Praise for
A Dude's Guide to Baby Size

"As a dad, I find the biggest gift another dad can give me is their honesty. The assignment of caring for another human being can be insanely daunting, and knowing that other dads, like Taylor, are dealing with the same stuff and able to encourage and joke about it is all I want to hear."

—TONY HALE, actor and comedian

"Your partner is pregnant? This book will guide you through the dos and don'ts, which will really cut down the number of times you hear, 'Remember when I was pregnant and you thought it was a good idea to . . . ?' *A Dude's Guide to Baby Size* will give you the perspective of a dad who's been there, done that—and his wife still loves him. Through his down-to-earth tone filled with humor, great anecdotes, and heartfelt advice, Taylor Calmus will help you make the most of what's guaranteed to be the most crazy, nerve-racking, and beautiful adventure of your entire life."

—KRISTINA KUZMIČ, speaker and author of
Hold On, But Don't Hold Still

"This is the book I needed fifteen years ago. New parenthood books scared the crap out of me, but Taylor's book gives me a warm, fuzzy feeling and helps me realize everything will be okay. It makes me want to have another baby, except there's nothing in the book about how to reverse a vasectomy."

—PENN HOLDERNESS, chief creative officer of
Holderness Family Productions and co-author of
Everybody Fights: So Why Not Get Better at It?

"Do you want to have a better understanding of what both mom and baby are going through during pregnancy? Taylor walks you through this journey in a way that not only helps a soon-to-be dad understand the logistics of pregnancy but also invites him into connecting with the baby before birth. He shares personal stories of parenting young children, lessons learned, and prompts to help you envision what it's going to be like to have the best title in the world: Dad. I'm super proud of Taylor and this book, and I'm not just saying that because he's my husband!"

—HEIDI CALMUS, wife and mother

A DUDE'S GUIDE TO BABY SIZE

A DUDE'S GUIDE TO BABY SIZE

WHAT TO EXPECT AND HOW TO PREP, FOR DADS-TO-BE

Taylor Calmus

WATERBROOK

No book can replace the diagnostic expertise and medical advice of a trusted physician. Please be certain to consult with your doctor before making any decisions that affect your health, particularly if you suffer from any medical condition or have any symptom that may require treatment.

Published in the United States by WaterBrook, an imprint of Random House, a division of Penguin Random House LLC.

WATERBROOK® and its deer colophon are registered trademarks of Penguin Random House LLC.

Library of Congress Cataloging-in-Publication Data
Names: Calmus, Taylor, author.
Title: A dude's guide to baby size : what to expect and how to prep for dads-to-be / by Taylor Calmus.
Description: Colorado Springs : WaterBrook, [2022] | Includes bibliographical references.
Identifiers: LCCN 2021061611 | ISBN 9780593194416 (hardcover) | ISBN 9780593194423 (ebook)
Subjects: LCSH: Pregnancy. | Fatherhood.
Classification: LCC RG551 .C35 2022 | DDC 618.2—dc23/eng/20220203
LC record available at https://lccn.loc.gov/2021061611

Printed in the United States of America on acid-free paper

waterbrookmultnomah.com

1st Printing

First Edition

Book design by Diane Hobbing

SPECIAL SALES Most WaterBrook books are available at special quantity discounts when purchased in bulk by corporations, organizations, and special-interest groups. Custom imprinting or excerpting can also be done to fit special needs. For information, please email specialmarketscms@penguinrandomhouse.com.

CONTENTS

Things She'll Say During the Second Trimester 45

Things She'll Say During the Third Trimester 101

Extras

INTRODUCTION

GENTLEMEN, START YOUR ENGINES

Well, you've done it—you've gotten your lady pregnant. *Boom. Nailed it!* Isn't it funny how you never know if your boys can swim until they do? Well, cheers to you, my friend. Your loins are home state to at least one squirmy little Olympian. If your wife gave you this book and you're confused right now, let me just say this one more time—

YOU ARE GOING TO BE A FATHER. CONGRATS!

In less than forty weeks, you'll be a pop holding your dear little offspring, but so much will happen between now and then. Your house will become cluttered with baby paraphernalia, your Corvette may get traded in for a Honda Odyssey, and your lady will gain a solid twenty to forty pounds. That's the equivalent of an average-sized house dog. But you know all that already! What you don't know is what is happening inside your wife's incubator—the womb. She surely has a few books comparing your unborn child to an apple or a stalk of broccoli, but I take issue with that. First off, your baby isn't some weenie little vegetable. Your baby is a hardcore little badass that is straight-up growing organs on a weekly basis. Second, how big is a stalk of broccoli? What the heck is a kumquat? Nope. No more. I introduce to you . . . *A Dude's Guide to Baby Size.*

Inside this book you'll find information on your growing baby, encouragement for helping Mom-to-be, and ideas for how to begin to become a Dude Dad. Each week's title, along with the corresponding image, is an example of what the baby's size is at that week—but the object is something a dad will know!

Now, I know guys don't like to be told how to do things; I don't either. It's why we don't stop for directions. I hate those videos of people telling parents the proper way to get their kids to poop or how to make a baby sleep for fourteen hours straight. Nobody's an expert on parenting. Okay, maybe you are if you have ten or more kids and they're all nuns, but otherwise, nope. You're just winging it. I know I'm not an expert. I've read only three books about parenting (and this is one of them). Plus, every kid is unique and wired differently. But have I gone through this? Yes. Can I tell you about my experiences and hope you'll learn something from them? Yeah, I can do that. I'll share my experiences and what has and hasn't worked for me. If you want to do it my way, cool. If you don't . . . well, good luck.

There are a lot of things a dad-to-be can do during pregnancy besides gaining more weight than the mom-to-be. You're starting an amazing journey right now, so I hope I can come along and help you through to the moment you hold your little lug nut for the very first time. Think of me as your best friend who is eager to help you prepare for what will be the biggest transition of your life. This book isn't necessarily about pregnancy; it's about fatherhood. Since these forty weeks are part of an incredible ride you're taking with your wife, these pages will help start to open you up to fatherhood.

Things She'll Say During the **First** Trimester

"You did this. You did this to me."

"Nothing fits. I'm too small for maternity clothes and too big for regular clothes . . . Guess it's a leggings day."

"Babe. You cannot let me eat after 6 P.M. anymore. No, I need you to pull your weight too. And that is watching mine."

(Twenty minutes later) "You do not get to tell me when I can and cannot eat. Are you carrying a child?"

"My body is making a baby. What is your body doing? Just sweating and growing hair."

"I have to pee. I have to pee. I have to pee. Oh my gosh, I have to pee. I have to pee."

"Babe, I feel so sick. I haven't been to Target in like four days. That's how sick I feel. Think I could be having withdrawals."

"Well, it's actually super healthy for pregnant women to fart, so you should just be happy that I'm healthy."

"Zzzzzzz."

"Babe, we need new shampoo. This scent makes me nauseous."

"Babe, my boobs are getting so big from all the extra hormones . . . Not those kinds of hormones. I have a headache."

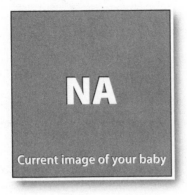

Current image of your baby

IT BEGINS

I know what you're thinking: *I don't see anything.* During this week, your little nugget isn't actually conceived yet. The lining of the uterus is thickening and preparing for guests. Your wife's uterus is like a bed-and-breakfast that's open only once a month. Even if nobody shows up, they still make the beds, wash the towels, and clean the waffle iron. And if the guests show up on the wrong date, they get sent packing. *Sorry, buddy—closed for renovations.* But your little dude knew that and won't be checking in till next week. He's just chilling out, waiting for construction to be complete. Baby made reservations. That's how hardcore your baby is. Sound like broccoli to you? Didn't think so.

So over these forty weeks, you're going to need to learn a lot about the female body and all the fantastic things it can do. Hey—if she can carry a baby and go into labor, is it too much to ask you to do a little homework? To give you a jump start on your gestation education, here are some important pregnancy words you need to know, dude-splained:

Chromosomes: Remember the mosquitoes in *Jurassic Park* that were encapsulated in the tree sap and carried the dino DNA? Basically that.

Ovaries: Think of these as gumball machines inside a woman that release one gumball (egg) a month into the hopper (fallopian tubes).

Embryo: For the first eight weeks, your fertilized egg doesn't have a name, so they came up with this one. But seriously. Who would want to be called Embryo? Imagine Embryo on the playground (cue the soundtrack of a Pixar film). Embryo is sliding down the fallopian tube, picking up all these cells before she enters the uterus.

Amniotic sac: This is the sac of fluid that your baby lives in inside the womb. It's like a Jacuzzi that is set to the perfect baby-growing temp, and your baby just chills in it for nine months.

Placenta: This is the organ that connects to the uterus and gives your growing baby everything he needs. Picture a personal chef next to your baby's hot tub who provides baby with the perfect nutrition plan throughout pregnancy.

Lamaze: A martial art practiced by ninjas in the mountains of Japan a thousand years ago.

Hyperemesis: Think of the worst hangover *ever*. But this kind of morning sickness comes from being pregnant and not from the case of Milwaukee's Best you had last night.

Booty bombs: This is just a warning that your wife is going to be farting. A lot.

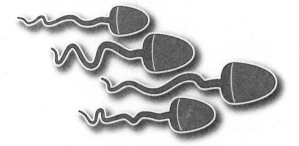

SPERM

Now is the time to enjoy lots of sex with your partner, so go for it—as often as you like.

—*PREGNANCY DAY BY DAY*

I second that.

—TAYLOR CALMUS

THIS IS SPARTA!

When you and your lady get to it, you release about 250 million sperm. This is like a freaking army of little white soldiers playing a game of Capture the Egg. Which is totally relevant because a vagina is basically a war zone filled with land mines and booby traps that kill off a ton of the sperm. This stuff is straight-up medieval. It's survival of the fittest, and most soldiers won't make it. Sometimes it ends in a literal bloodbath, aka the period. (Come on, man—don't get grossed out now. If you're going to make it as a dad, you're going to need a stronger stomach.)

In the movie *300*, King Leonidas leads three hundred Spartans in battle against Xerxes and his army. In your epic movie, only about two hundred of 250 million sperm arrive at the site of the egg. Despite all the odds, your strongest little soldier breaks through the castle walls and conquers the egg.

Boom.

Sparks. Magic. Pixie dust.

CONCEPTION.

SO YOU'RE TELLING ME THERE'S A CHANCE

Did you know sperm have less than a 1 in 1,000,000 chance of making it to the place of fertilization? That is *insane* odds. You're more likely to be killed by flesh-eating bacteria than a sperm is to reach fertilization. In fact, here's a list of ridiculous things that are more likely to happen.

You have a 1 in 662,000 chance of winning an Olympic gold medal.

You have a 1 in 11,500 chance of winning an Academy Award.

You have a 1 in 250,000 chance of getting killed by a meteorite.

You have a 1 in 500 chance of being born with eleven fingers or toes.

And you have a 1 in 10,000 chance of being injured by a toilet.

The good news is that you don't have just one sperm to bet on. You're at the horse races, and you've got a good feeling about Western Showdown, but you're also going to throw down a bet on about 250 million other horses as well. All you need is one horse to win.

Let's call him Lucky Strike.

OVULATION 101

Let's talk about the mystery of the female body: Ovulation.

Ovulation occurs once a month when an egg moves from one of the ovaries down the fallopian tube and into the uterus. It's there that it waits for twelve to twenty-four hours to be fertilized by sperm. If it's not fertilized, it passes out through menstruation.

So you might be thinking, *As long as we don't have intercourse during ovulation, she can't get pregnant.*

False.

Let me explain by metaphor.

Imagine that your wife's uterus is Best Buy and this Best Buy is open only one day a month. They have a sale item, something that everybody wants: a PS5 (or whatever version they're selling when you're reading this book). So people don't show up just on the day of the sale. Sometimes they'll show up three or five days in advance and they'll just wait around, like in a tent or with a sandwich, or maybe they'll peruse a magazine, or maybe they'll make friends with another person and decide to go in together.

Most of the sperm are like your slacker friends from college who give up waiting for the PS5 and go home early. But finally ovulation starts and the remaining sperm bull-rush into the Best Buy, looking for the PS5. It's like those crazy videos you see online of Black Friday free-for-alls. Some of them just get lost in the TV and home theater department. They're like, *Look at that ... Is that a seventy-five-inch screen? That's pretty slick.* Then the lucky ones will find the PS5. Fertilization starts, a baby is conceived, and the pregnancy begins.

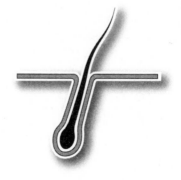

HAIR FOLLICLE

Have you ever shaved early in the morning and then spent all day out and about interacting with people only to get home and realize that you missed a very obvious little patch of facial hair and have looked like a moron all day? Well, you're not a moron. You're just . . . busy. But your baby is currently the size of one of those hair follicles, and like that lone follicle, your baby is undetected. You and your lady have just been living like normal, not knowing that your baby exists.

You probably also don't know that your baby already has forty-six chromosomes that determine his or her hair color, eye color, body type, and ability to grow and forget about things like facial hair. Out of those forty-six chromosomes, one from you and one from your wife determine the sex of your baby. During this period, your developing baby will reach the uterus, and magical things will begin to happen. He or she is going to be one of a kind with details like no other.

At this point you don't even know that your little biscuit is now his own unique piece of art with his own set of fingerprints. Those fingerprints will someday be on everything he touches that defines who he is and the impact he'll have on the world. Maybe your kid will wield an ice pick while scaling Mt. Everest, or maybe he'll sit at a computer, hacking the mainframe of North Korea to prevent a nuclear attack. One place those fingerprints will definitely be is on the sliding glass door in your house . . . right next to all the slobber marks and smears. Regardless, the adventure is just beginning—and you don't even know you're on one!

WHAT'S THE STORY, MORNING GLORY?

From one dude to another, here's something you need to know right away: Morning sickness is a lie. Mama's nausea is gonna come anytime it wants. In the middle of the day or night. And even if you think you can't do a thing about it, think again. There are lots of things you can do to help with this not-so-fun part of being pregnant:

1. Be sensitive. Most guys aren't the best with this particular trait, but if you're reading this book, chances are you're different. This leads to my second suggestion . . .
2. Don't make jokes. Okay, I know—that's what I do for a living. But when your lady is clinging to the toilet bowl for dear life, it's no time to be doing your best Jim Gaffigan bit.
3. Eliminate odors. This is definitely hard since you're a dude. But think before you douse yourself with Axe body spray. Don't put Limburger cheese on your burger. Keep your stanky socks away from her.

4. Give her encouragement, not exhortation. I doubt you're a doctor, and that's okay because neither am I. Tell her she's doing great, and when you can't think of anything good to say, try number 5.
5. Stay silent. Sometimes it's good to just zip it up.

BB

Your little bean has finally made her way down the fallopian tube and implanted in the uterus. Baby is about the size of one BB right now, which doesn't seem like much, but remember it takes only one BB to the head to take down a twenty-four-pound turkey. Little one isn't even out of the gestational sac, and she's already bringing home dinner—what a rock star.

When you think of BB guns, it's easy to picture Ralphie from *A Christmas Story* finally getting the holy grail of Christmas gifts, an official Red Ryder carbine-action, two-hundred-shot, range-model air rifle. He carefully holds it for the first time, marveling at its beauty and feeding it with BBs. It's a dream come true. Becoming a father for the first time is just like opening that Christmas present you've been dreaming about for your entire life. But with this gift comes a huge responsibility.

A BB gun is a symbol of trust. When I was seven years old, my parents entrusted me with one. My dad is big into hunting, so he spent a lot of time teaching me how to use my BB gun, showing me the proper safety protocol, the visual and physical checks to ensure that the weapon was unloaded before I took it into the house. He drilled gun safety into my siblings and me to the point where we knew that a gun wasn't something to mess around with.

My dad trusting me with the BB gun made me want to be trustworthy, unlike Ralphie in *A Christmas Story*. After being warned over and over again that he could shoot his eye out, he finally gets his present and (spoiler alert) nearly does exactly that, breaking his glasses in the process and then straight-up lying to his mom about it.

I have my own Christmas story. I once got my head caught in an elevator.

Let me explain.

When I was a kid, I spent a lot of time playing on my uncles' farm. My uncles are very creative guys. If something doesn't exist, they just make it. They had this massive shop where they worked on all their tractors and farm equipment, and it had a big catwalk where they stored parts and miscellaneous other stuff up high and out of the way. Instead of having stairs to get up to the catwalk, they built an elevator out of angle iron. Picture an open-frame box with no walls. A cable connected the top of this box to a motor.

My cousin and I were instructed *not* to play on the elevator . . . so that is exactly what we did. One day when we had been left alone, we were screwing around like ten-year-old boys do, pressing the button to go up and down the makeshift elevator. I was at the top, starting to descend, when I got the idiotic idea to jump back onto the platform. The elevator was already too low, though, so I didn't make it all the way. Instead, I was just hanging on to the edge of the catwalk, with only my hands and my chin sticking just above it.

The cage of the elevator lowered onto the back of my neck, pinching me between the catwalk and the top of the elevator frame. The thing was pretty heavy but, thank God, not heavy enough to just cut me in two. My cousin, who was the same size as me, was underneath the elevator, trying to lift it off me. The only reason I survived was that the motor hadn't hit its trip point at the bottom, so all the cable unspooled, then wound back up the other way, lifting the elevator frame off me.

You can imagine the sort of mark the elevator made on my neck.

"Okay, Lincoln," I told my cousin. "We gotta come up with a lie."

His dad had all this junk behind the shop, so we decided to say we were playing back there and then I tripped and fell and hit my neck on something. Perfect story. It's Uncle Mike's fault. Clean up your junk, Uncle Mike! I figured we would go inside and lie just like Ralphie did in *A Christmas Story*. My parents totally bought it (I mean, I thought they did). Yet when I went to school the next day, guilt started eating me alive.

So when my dad picked me up after school, I decided to tell him the truth. Well . . . draw him the truth. As a kid, I was known for being a pretty good artist, so I sketched my parents a picture of me with my head stuck in the elevator. What kind of kid does this? Imagine your kid handing you *a picture* explaining how he lied. "Here's an illustration of my lie, Dad. This is what happened and my conscience can't take it. So I penciled this illustration to make sure you understand precisely how I lied."

I couldn't lie to my parents. At a very young age, they had shown me they trusted me, so knowing I had broken their trust ended up breaking my heart.

As fathers, we're going to have to trust our kids enough for them to go out and make mistakes, hoping that they'll come to us and tell us when they mess up. The worst thing that can happen is for our kids to hide things from us because they're afraid of our (over)reaction. Not that they shouldn't get in big trouble, but we want them to trust us enough to let us know what's really going on. That way we can help them try to fix whatever got broken. Giving our kids a little trust can help them learn to be trustworthy.

TEN THINGS I LEARNED ABOUT BABIES IN THE FIRST YEAR

1. They Don't Cry as Much as You'd Think

Unless you have a colicky baby, it's really not that bad. Before kids, you might hear that piercing cry from someone else's kiddo and say, "Oh my gosh, will you just take its batteries out?" But after you have a kid, you sort of just get used to it. Then again, maybe we've just had really good babies.

2. They Don't Cost as Much as You'd Think

Don't get me wrong—there are expenses, but everybody makes it sound like it's going to bankrupt you. I'm sure it will add up over time, but for the first year, not so much. Most of what they eat is boob food. If you have a baby shower, people will buy you most of the stuff, and whatever you don't have, just network with other parents and they'll happily give away their kids' stuff. "Do you want to take this swing too?"

3. You'll Learn to Function with Less Sleep

At first it's awful getting up one, two, or twenty-seven times a night, especially when you're a sleep connoisseur like me. I prefer to get between eight and ten hours of sleep every night. But I can barely remember what that feels like. A few years into this thing, and you'll realize you're absolutely crushing it despite all the wake-ups. You'll be like, *Dang, look at all this stuff I got done with only five hours of sleep!*

4. You Can't Keep Living like You Did

Before we were parents, our friends had a baby. I remember always thinking, *Why don't they just bring him with?* Now I know why. So just adjust and be honest. "Yeah . . . No, sorry. We can't come tonight." Which leads to my next point . . .

5. You'll Use Your Baby as an Excuse Whenever You Can

"Sorry I'm late for work . . . my baby."

"I planned on going to the gym today, but . . . my baby."

"I planned on making dinner tonight, but . . . my baby."

"I couldn't get on the Zoom call because—you know—my baby."

"Sorry I was driving so fast, Officer. It's just, my baby . . ."

"I know I forgot your birthday, but . . . my baby."

"I would love to come to your one-man show, but . . . even my baby knows how painful one-man shows are."

6. Babies Evolve—Fast

The minute you think you got your baby figured out—whether it be sleeping, eating habits, whatever—boom. She changes completely.

7. You'll See Your Partner in a Whole New Light

Parenting brings out parts of you that you didn't know were there. You can observe this in your partner. For instance, Heidi is a bear cat. There have been several occasions when completely for no reason she has said, "If anyone ever hurts our children, I will kill them." And she says it in a way that makes me not want to ask questions. On the flip side, when she sees me with the kids, she describes me as "a playful kitten." So that's something.

8. You'll See Your Parents in a Whole New Light

As a kid or even as a young adult, you can't really grasp everything your parents did for you. Then you have a kid, and suddenly you realize everything you must have put them through. You'll call your parents and just be like, "Sorry." They'll be like, "For what?"

"ALL OF IT."

9. Unsolicited Parenting Advice Is the Worst

"Your baby should really be wearing socks."

"You're really going to let your baby play with that?"

"You're not co-sleeping? You're a bad parent. You need to co-sleep so he can feel your warmth at night."

"You're not letting her cry it out? You're a bad parent. You need to let her cry it out so she's not a softie when she grows up."

Stop. Just stop. I'm sorry, random lady at Pep Boys. I don't care what you think about bottle-feeding. Just get your wiper fluid and then BEAT IT.

10. You'll Understand Love in a Whole New Way

This is the top thing I learned about babies in my first year. As humans, we're wired to look out for ourselves, but when you have a baby, he's an extension of yourself. A smaller, cuter version of yourself. On some days, he'll make you late for work and spill juice on your laptop and smear his own feces on the wall, reminding you that love is not just a feeling but an action. Then he'll reach up with his little hands and look into your eyes, and you'll feel it. No, not feces—thankfully. Love. Unconditional love.

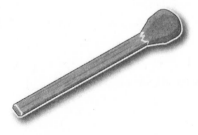

MATCH HEAD

Your match-head-sized child is now rapidly growing a spinal cord, heart, and blood vessels. It all started with a single spark, but then like a wildfire of joy, this baby is about to consume your world in the best way possible. You may be scared of all the changes coming, but did you know that some species of trees are actually fire dependent? Wildfires burn off vegetation, creating the right environment for some seeds to sprout. Without fire, these trees would eventually succumb to old age with no new generations to carry on their legacy.

Dude, that's so deep.

Imagine a tiny spark developing into a minuscule baby brain. So much is being formed inside your baby right now. The first heartbeats occur twenty-one days after conception, so it's time to start preparing for your own heart to expand with wonder and joy.

Speaking of sparks, chances are there might not be a lot between you and your lady. She has likely been slapping your hands away, as her body is going through rapid changes and her breasts are becoming extremely tender. She's also getting fatigued easily. Don't take offense, though—a tiny human has made her uterus into a guest bedroom, and we all know how draining it can be to entertain guests. Especially when your guest is depending on you for all her nutrition and well-being. Dang. At least you don't have to make small talk the whole time.

So just in case you've been living in the Dark Ages, let me shine a light on another symptom that your wife will be experiencing very soon if she isn't already. Mood swings. She might suddenly cry for no reason, and the next moment she might sound completely irrational. This time, it's probably not your fault. You can blame those raging hormones inside her. But also, a word to the wise: Maybe don't blame those hormones out loud. Keep that one to yourself.

TAKE HEART

Pregnancy is super exciting, but it can also be scary, and when things take an unexpected turn, it can be really tough.

I asked Heidi if it would be okay for me to share one of our week 5 stories with you guys, but before I do, let me just say this—if you've ever lost a pregnancy, you're not alone . . .

During our first pregnancy, right around week 5, Heidi woke up in the middle of the night, saying something didn't feel right. She went to the bathroom, and when she came back with tears in her eyes, she told me we had lost the baby. It felt unreal. I did everything I could to comfort her. We went back to bed, held each other tight, and tried to sleep, but with little avail. In the morning I woke up wondering if it had really happened. Was it some sort of bad dream? But sadly, it had happened. Unfortunately, it's happened to lots of couples out there, and thankfully, we had some friends to walk through this with us. If you've ever lost a pregnancy, I'd encourage you to find some trusted friends or family members to share your journey with. It's a tough thing to walk through alone, and the likelihood is that others in your circle have walked through it as well.

As a guy, I felt a sense of hurt and loss, even though I hadn't met our little one. I had just barely found out that we were pregnant. So I lost what I thought was going to come, a vision of the future, as if my front-row concert tickets had just gotten canceled. But for Heidi, this was a little person she had literally felt inside her body, a piece of her—and now that piece was gone. It's important to process your own experience of loss while also being present to your lady, who is going to need you in a big way.

A lot of couples I know who have kids have also experienced a miscarriage along the way. At week 5, the chance of a miscarriage is around 20 percent. This drops dramatically by week 14, when there is less than a 1 percent chance of a miscarriage. If this isn't your family's story, I'm not trying to invite unnecessary worry—largely the stats are on your side. If this is your family's story, you aren't alone.

Take heart, my friends. There is much to hope for . . . Three months later, we got pregnant again, and nine months after that, we had our son Theo. My suspicion is that since you hold this book in your hands, there is much to celebrate in the present, and the future is bright. Take heart! And help other dads do the same.

I wrote this piece for Heidi on her first-ever Mother's Day.

MY SON'S MOM

My son's mom is a badass. Not in the traditional sense.

No.

She doesn't wear camo
or carry a gun with lots of ammo.

She is smiley and gracious and diffuses lavender on a very regular
basis.

My son's mom is a badass in how she **loves.**

She is full-metal-jacket, hug-you-till-you're-blue,
jump-in-front-of-a-bus-for-you LOVE.

Her love for our son has changed her in ways that not only make
me proud but make me laugh. The other day, pushing the stroller
across the street, a car screams by within a few feet, and for the first
time, she threw her finger in the air, yelling, "HEY! THERE'S A
BABY HERE!"

My son's mom.
She is a lion, a viper.
"YOU MESS WITH HIM AND I WILL CUT YOU!"

I fear for the someone someday that picks on our son.

As his father, I will teach him self-defense while all the while teaching
him how to use his words, not his hands. But my son's mom . . .

She. Will. Crush you.

It will be no contest—there will be no second chances.

She will rip out your throat and shove it in your pants.

My son's mom.

I love my son, but I would be lying if I didn't mention that I
thought him a stranger the first time I met him.

He looks like me—
that I see.
But we have no history.

You see, I became a father when we made our first connection.
But my son's mom, she knew him from a whole other dimension.

She knew him from long ago
inside her womb starting to grow.
She knew him before she even began to show.

Little kicks, sleeping habits.
Can we get some Oreos? Baby needs his fix!

See, she became a mom when they made their first connection,
which for her was at conception.
Except that's not even right, because there's something else I haven't
mentioned.

You see, three months before, we had another blessing,
a faint blue line that kept us guessing.
A baby?
Maybe.

And then two days later, we had confirmation
that, yes indeed, it was gestation.
I am going to be a father!

But it wasn't long and something felt wrong.

And five weeks in, our baby was gone.

People told us it happens more often than you'd think.

Now, I don't mean to be dramatic, but a lot of people get cancer
too.
Does that make that any less tragic?

This is a baby that I never knew.
But my son's mom knew him and felt him too.

So today I want to honor her strength
because I have now seen it in length.

A mother's love is AUTHENTIC,
RELENTLESS
ACCEPTANCE.

I write this piece because my son is too young to express it.
But every word is confirmed in his contentment.

She is the bomb.
She is my son's mom.

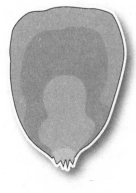

KERNEL OF POPCORN

At six weeks, your little partner is currently the size of a kernel of popcorn.

Remember when you first heard you were going to be a dad? Do you recall the moments before that pivotal revelation?

There you were, oblivious to this tiny object in your wife's belly. While that bump wouldn't be showing for a while, she was experiencing lots of growth and changes deep inside her—like your baby's heart. It was developing quickly and starting to pump blood, just like yours started to when you got the big news!

Just like a hard kernel popping into the soft goodness that is popcorn, the news of your baby suddenly expanded your whole life. Everything changed in a split second. Your jaw dropped to the ground while you tried to understand what this meant. You didn't know how to collect yourself. Maybe you gave a nervous laugh or even shed a few tears.

One second, and boom—you're going to be a father. And you're going to *change*.

And before you go thinking that your wife is the only one whose body is about to change, think again. Science now says that a "love hormone" called oxytocin not only helps mothers bond with their children but also increases in fathers when they hold their newborns. This oxytocin racing through a father lowers his testosterone while increasing another hormone—prolactin. This is the hormone that helps fill women with breast milk. Experts don't say men are going to be breastfeeding anytime soon, but prolactin helps fathers play with their children in better ways.

What? You didn't think that being responsible for *another human walking and breathing on this planet* was going to affect you? You now have the amazing gift of being not just a provider but a teacher, a guide, and a protector. Maybe you've always seen yourself as Luke Skywalker, but now you can be Obi-Wan Kenobi, Yoda, and Chewbacca too! It's your turn to guide a young Padawan.

COMING ATTRACTIONS

So imagine you're in a theater, holding a jumbo-sized tub of popcorn drenched with ten pumps of "butter" as you watch all the previews. Now, what sort of movie trailer do you picture for your life as a parent? What sort of story do you want your life to tell once your little dude or dudette arrives?

Maybe the trailer shows you a movie you don't think you're ready for. Because, for some people, finding out they're pregnant is a giant shift in their life plans.

But I was planning on moving to Florida to pursue a career as a beach-stand airbrush artist.

Maybe hold off on that dream for a beat. It doesn't have to go away forever, but you're going to need to get your feet back under you.

Wait a minute. Does this mean I have to stop making meth with my old chemistry teacher from Albuquerque?

Um . . . yes.

That is a "dream" you should probably put on pause—and never pick back up. For sooo many reasons.

Every pregnancy story is its own genre. For our first, it was a coming-of-age story. Our second child was a rom-com because it was like, "Oh no, here we go!" Then the third one was probably more of a suspense film, a story building and building with all this pressure. Your pregnancy might be something different. Maybe neither of you has any idea how you got pregnant in the first place, which puts you squarely in the science-fiction genre.

It doesn't matter what genre your pregnancy feels like so far. The good news is that you have the ability to influence the eventual film, to direct that story. You have control over the production of that movie called *Becoming a Family.*

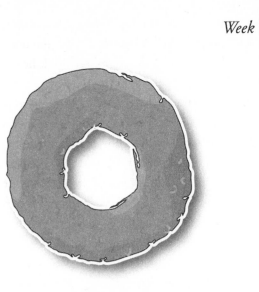

CHEERIO

Ch-ch-ch-ch-changes. This week, a mouth and tongue are starting to be defined. Upper and lower buds are growing into arms and legs. A brain that will one day be way smarter than yours is becoming more complex.

Mom-to-be is changing as well. Mood swings. Worry about weight. Happy-sad fluctuations that can make Dad feel like he's walking on a tightrope. Don't worry. Don't panic. And don't take it personally. Instead, just shut up and try to be helpful.

CHEERIOHHS

Your baby is now the size of a Cheerio, and if you can't picture this, well, be prepared to. My household has already gone through no less than three truckloads of Cheerios. We eat so many Cheerios in this house, I find them everywhere. They're on the floor. They're under the couch. They're in my car. They're in my shoes. There are so many

Cheerios around our house, my dog won't even eat them anymore. When our kids spill their Cheerios, I point the dog at 'em, but he just gives me a look of *Nah, I'm good.* I think he's holding out for Lucky Charms.

So what makes this bland cereal so endearing to parents? Maybe it's because they're dry and don't get stuck on anything. They don't make a big mess—you just vacuum them up after you step on them. They're easy for babies to pick up, and they dissolve in those tiny, toothless mouths.

Cheerios are boring but efficient. They're something to help parents get their kids through the day without a meltdown at the bank.

Picture it now. Your baby is strapped in his high chair, and you give him a few Cheerios, and he's playing with them, and you're just getting through the day. Time goes by, and now your little Tater Tot has one of those cups with the lid that he can open and shove his hand inside to take out some Cheerios. He enjoys this snack as he runs errands with you, and you're just getting through the day. Soon he's a bit older, and you're giving him a bowl of Cheerios with milk before preschool. He's spilling half of it, but that's okay because you're just getting through the day. And before you know it, he's a teenager, and he's pouring his own bowl of Cheerios, and you barely see him do it, and you're still just getting through the day.

Cheerios are the flavorless little things that just help you get through the day. You don't have time to stop and appreciate every single Cheerio, but at some point it's going to be just you and your wife sitting there with a box of stale Cheerios, and the kids will be gone. And now you're eating them because your cholesterol is too high.

Here's the truth: Those mundane moments matter just like Cheerios. They might seem bland when you're going through them, but one day you'll look back and say, "Remember when the kids were teething? Remember when we used to sit at the table and stare at them while they ate their food because that was the only way they would eat? When was the last time I watched my kid eat? When was the last time I gave him that much attention at the dinner table?"

We often don't think about these things in the moment. But later on, simply making it through the monotony that parenting can be will bring memories you treasure. So don't discount those Cheerio moments. One day they'll matter more than you can ever know.

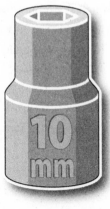

TEN-MILLIMETER SOCKET

FUN FACT

Here's something that will blow your mind: Your baby's brain is currently growing at 250,000 cells per minute. The arms, the legs, the head—everything is expanding! Those tiny limbs are starting to twitch, but Mommy won't feel this. Not yet.

NOT-SO-FUN FACT

Mommy is starting to feel the changes inside her body. Her stomach is feeling tight, and that's not just because of that bucket of chicken she ate last night at KFC. Just like the baby, her uterus is growing—it will eventually become five hundred times as big as it used to be. Something else that might be growing? Her mood swings. Oh yeah, they're going to start swinging from the rooftops. Imagine PMS on steroids. Or imagine steroids with PMS? I'm not sure which. I've never had either, but it's a lot at once.

She might still be experiencing morning sickness. The weird thing is that she can get morning sickness in the afternoon or right before bed. I bet some dude coined the phrase. "Nah, you're not really feelin' morning sickness, babe. That's only after you wake up." Maybe it should just be called baby sickness? Who knows? But like Batman, it can strike at a moment's notice.

Your little dude is now the size of a ten-millimeter socket. "What size is this?" you might ask. It's the one socket you can imagine. This is the socket that you use the most, and it's the one that's often missing since it's always being taken out of the toolbox. When you're working on cars, for instance, there are lots of places where a ten-millimeter socket is needed. Since you're constantly using it, it's going to be misplaced. Not lost, but simply left somewhere. So you're always on the hunt for this ten-millimeter socket.

In the parenting world, the ten-millimeter socket is the pacifier. People call this wonderful invention many things—the paci, soother, binky, boo-ba, nuker, nuk, or nukie.

I prefer to call it the nukie. You use it in the living room, the nursery, the bedroom, the park, the car . . . *everywhere.* When you need it, it's not always where it's supposed to be, so you have to go looking for it.

Some babies don't like the nuk, but others *love* it, so when you lose it, the baby loses her mind. Let me paint you a nightmarish picture starring the nukie.

You're home alone with your baby, and she's already been fed, but she's starting to get fussy. You've swaddled her and put her on her back in her crib, but now she's crying. You hold her and shush her, but the crying gets louder, so you sway and swing her. She only gets more angry, wailing now. You realize you need the nukie, but the nukie is nowhere to be found. So you begin to tear the house apart.

You try to remember where you had it, but you can't, so you start backtracking. You check the bedroom, then the nursery. You go out and look in your car and the car seat. You check the diaper bag, then decide to go back upstairs to check under your bed. You look in the dishwasher and under the couch. All the while you're holding a seemingly demon-possessed child who is roaring in all her fury. You're forced to call your wife, who is out with her girlfriends. She tells you there's another pack of nukies on the top shelf of the cupboard just left of the stove. So you leave the screaming baby in her bouncy seat, crawl on top of the counter, open the cupboard full of scented candles and cookbooks, then finally find the pack and pull one out. You can't believe how long this took, but *you did it all for the nukie.*

Yes, I wrote all that just to make this Limp Bizkit joke, but it's still a valid point.

Like a ten-millimeter socket, a pacifier is easy to lose. So buy a couple of packs, and put them everywhere.

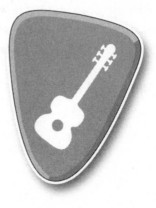

GUITAR PICK

Your little shredder is the size of the flat surface of a guitar pick and is rocking out at about 150 heartbeats per minute. Only nine weeks old, and listen to that rhythm! Eat your heart out, Travis Barker. Your baby is now putting on sold-out womb shows for you and your doctor. Also, is it just me, or are the acoustics in this uterus fantastic?

Take some time to come up with a clever band name for your unborn child like UltraSoundgarden, Tom Petty and the Heartbeaters, or my wife's favorite, My Morning Sickness. I hear they do amazing covers from Nirvana's *In Utero*. I'm having wwwway too much fun right now. But seriously, jot your band name right here in the margin!

Even though your baby can't hear Foo Fighters blasting from your Bose speakers (that comes around week 18), tiny indentations are forming that will eventually become ears. Fingers that might one day shred a Fender Stratocaster are becoming more distinct. His oversize noggin is bent down, as if he's preparing to one day be a headbanger—hopefully the fun kind like in *Wayne's World*.

What sort of songs would you like to play for your son or daughter one day? Make a list of tunes to play while baby is still in the womb. Or make a fun assortment of tracks for your wife. Here's an example of a playlist that tells the tale of days to come . . .

PLAYLIST FOR PREGNANT PARENTS

For her midnight cravings . . .
"Pour Some Sugar on Me" by Def Leppard

When she has to go pee . . .
"Wake Me Up Before You Go-Go" by Wham!

When she feels the baby for the first time . . .
"Whoomp! There It Is" by Tag Team

When the baby keeps kicking . . .
"Jump Around" by House of Pain

When she asks if she looks fat . . .
"Baby Got Back" by Sir Mix-A-Lot

For morning sickness . . .
"You Spin Me Round (like a Record)" by Dead or Alive

Your wife and sex during the first trimester . . .
"Love Lockdown" by Kanye West

Your wife during the second trimester . . .
"Let's Get It On" by Marvin Gaye

When she's struggling with her body image . . .
"Your Body Is a Wonderland" by John Mayer

How to deal with her mood swings . . .
"Enjoy the Silence" by Depeche Mode

When someone's freaking out about becoming a parent . . .
"You Need to Calm Down" by Taylor Swift

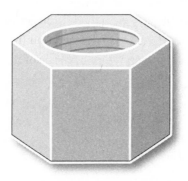

LUG NUT

Baby dude is now the size of a lug nut, and it's time for you, like a lug nut, to hold your sh** together. Your lady is starting to have some serious mood swings, and if you're not careful, you could end up on the chopping block. It'll be in your best interest to try to think before you speak—I mean, that's true most days, but just don't do what I did. I made the mistake of telling my wife that it was okay that her butt was getting big, because it was like our baby had a two-stall garage. In my head it was a compliment—I'd freaking *kill* to have a two-stall garage at my house. Anyway, if thinking before you speak is an issue for you, maybe just go mow the lawn or clean out the garbage disposal. Or better yet, paint the baby's room.

In your baby, all sorts of things are being formed like bones and knees and a nose. Mechanics are being tested for the first time, like bending at the wrists. The head is becoming rounder, and the eyes are shifting to a more central place on the face.

As much as the baby is changing, so is Mommy. Her body is going through *lots*. For guys, this is always hard to understand, other than seeing the extra curves. So picture pregnancy as something else. Imagine that your wife is a sleek and sexy red Ford F-150 that is being converted into a monster truck.

The first noticeable differences are the bigger tires (boobs) on the truck and the larger front and rear suspension (belly). But that's just the start. It's what's happening on the inside of the truck that makes it truly incredible. Putting in a supercharger (umbilical cord) increases the pressure of air entering the engine (placenta) in order to provide more oxygen (oxygen). Of course, a monster truck needs a roll cage (amniotic sac) to protect its passenger (baby).

Now that the F-150 has been transformed into a monster truck, you're going to notice more changes. The monster truck takes more gas, which is ironic because your wife will have lots more gas as well. You're going to have to make a lot more pit stops, just like your wife is going to be needing more potty breaks. The monster truck will occasionally be hard to crank (fatigue), and it will need to be taken to a mechanic (doctor) more often.

So if your lady is an F-150 turned into a monster truck, what are you?

You're a lug nut. Not all the lug nuts. You're a single lug nut. She's going to carry the weight of the entire pregnancy. It's your job to be there to support her and help hold everything together.

During this pregnancy, your wife is going to get sick and become tired and cranky. Maybe it's best to just stay out of her way right now. But she can also use your help (and, no, that doesn't mean just telling her to walk it off). She's doing everything to carry this baby to term, but you're also there, so why not do *something*? You can be a lug nut. Of course, she's also all the other lug nuts, but you can do your part and be one.

What if one of the lug nuts falls out of the vehicle? That's okay—she'll keep driving. But the wheel is going to spin a lot more easily if all the lug nuts are in there. You're there to help her along the journey, so do your part. Do whatever little things you can. If you don't, well, she's going to be fine because she's already doing everything. But maybe you can be one part of the process. You're just a small part of this supercharged monster truck, but you're an important part nevertheless.

THINGS NOT TO SAY TO
YOUR PREGNANT WIFE

"Babe, why did you buy another bra?"

"Babe? Are you peeing again? Are you seriously peeing again? Wow . . . Is your body like 100 percent urine right now?"

"I don't get why we need a crib and a Pack 'n Play."

"So you've just been sitting there eating pickles all day?"

"Babe, it's probably pregnancy brain. I just have to remember that you're not always like this."

(After she tells you she wants to go to Olive Garden) "Babe. I don't think you should eat carbs right now."

"I can build a crib from the scrap wood in the garage. It's just like a birdcage but bigger."

"I'm saying you're so small, you don't want the baby to be too big, because he'll just rip you open."

"Can we please find a cheaper belly balm?"

"Huh, your hips look different. Do you think they'll go back?"

"Is two weeks after the due date too soon for me to go on a camping trip? I already booked it."

"So what's up with your nipples?"

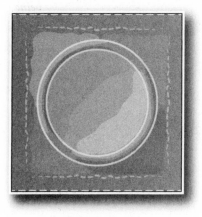

CONDOM

This is ironic. Your baby is now the size of that condom you didn't use. Awkward . . . Just kidding! Whether you and your lady planned this or not, you're going to be a father and it's going to be awesome. Crazy. But awesome. Know what else is awesome? Your baby is actually starting to look like a baby. She's got tiny hands and feet now and even ears. Yeah. *Ears.* You hear that? That's the sound of stuff getting real.

LET'S TALK ABOUT SEX, BABY

So let's be honest . . . Chances are you haven't been getting any "fun time" lately. Your wife's body is sort of like your favorite theme park. It has all your favorite rides, and the bosom mountain roller coaster just got a huge upgrade, so you're probably trying to get tickets right about now. Unfortunately, your wife's theme park will be running on limited hours for the next few months. And after birth, it will be closed for renovations for *six whole weeks.*

Take heart, my friend. This is the first trimester—your wife is dealing with fatigue and nausea and *a living being growing inside her belly that could one day become the president.* So just be patient. Get creative. The good news is that things might turn around for the better in the second trimester when the park is open, the lines are short, and the cotton candy is all free. And enjoy that while it lasts, because as the baby gets bigger and your wife becomes more uncomfortable, her sex drive is probably going to drop again in the third trimester. But all women are different, so you never know.

As a reminder, visiting the theme park right now is safe. Your sledgehammer isn't going to break down any walls, despite how hefty it might be. Your baby is secure in the uterus. I don't know *exactly* how it works, but I did look into it, and there is zero chance you can accidentally poke the baby. You're cool. Game on.

SO THIS WEEK . . .

- Tell your wife she's beautiful (without wanting to have sex).
- Give your wife a back rub (without wanting to have sex).
- Talk to your wife about your feelings about becoming a father.
- Ask your wife about her hopes and dreams for being a mom.
- Help out. Pitch in. Take the lead. Go ahead and do it. (Not because you want sex.)
- Read a book on pregnancy . . . Oh wait. You're already doing that. (You deserve sex.)

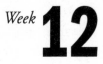

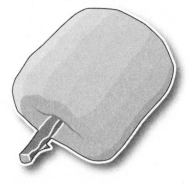

JUMBO MARSHMALLOW

Week 12 is a time to celebrate! The first trimester is coming to an end, so what better way to represent your baby than with a jumbo marshmallow? Marshmallows mean something fun is happening, whether you're making s'mores at a campfire or sipping hot chocolate in a horse-drawn sleigh or snacking on Rice Krispies Treats with your family. Maybe you're firing your marshmallow blaster or building a marshmallow tower. Whatever is happening, it's surely better than something involving meatloaf and *way* more exciting than eating mutton.

Your baby is celebrating, too, by waving his arms and legs. How do you know? It's because you can *see this with your own eyes*! Right around now, you get to have your first ultrasound scan, which is something you've been waiting for. This week is also a big milestone because the risk of having a miscarriage drops significantly.

So congratulations! You made it. This may or may not be your first time here, but it always feels good.

Naturally it's a great time to start sharing the good news. So go ahead, send out that group text! Or maybe brainstorm those pregnancy announcement ideas!

Do you put a bun in the oven for your family to find? How about announcing it with balloons or by wrapping up a baby onesie for your parents to open? You two can wear matching shirts sharing the news! Or wait . . . Get your dog to announce it in some way!

Now, just wait a minute. Let's not get too far ahead of ourselves here.

There are some things you'll want to consider before making the announcement. Once you tell people you're expecting, they'll start expecting to come on that journey with you. They'll ask questions every time you see them, some will also start giving you unsolicited advice, and some will even start touching your wife's stomach like it's a totally normal thing to do—usually without asking her. So do you really want *everyone* to know right away?

One definite thing to do, Dad: Make sure your wife knows who you're telling and when you're going to tell them.

PREGNANCY FEARS

Fears are natural during pregnancy. Especially with your first.

When we were having Theo, we were freaked out about everything, having gone through a miscarriage only months before getting pregnant with him. That had us more on edge, googling every question and concern while we held our breath. During our second pregnancy, however, we were more preoccupied and busy, which was probably good since we didn't have as much free time to worry. But then we got a call.

Around week 14, we went for a screening test where they did a blood draw to run a whole bunch of tests. If anything showed up, they would call us, and sure enough, that's what happened. Suddenly

Heidi and I found ourselves in some sort of suspense movie with the anxiety building and building.

The next day we went to see the doctor. We signed in and took our seats in the waiting room, where we waited and waited. Then they finally called our name and took us to another room with a table holding just a box of tissues. That was all—just the box of tissues. *Well, what the H-E-double-hockey-sticks is that for? Why did they sit us at a table with just a box of tissues? Why do we need tissues?* The specialist came in, and we braced ourselves for her to just lay the news on us, but instead, we were bombarded with questions. We had to go through our entire family history to see if there were any issues on either side. Basically just going through the ways our family members have died, which really brightened the mood. Then she pulled out a giant folder and shared the lab results that were concerning, talking about AFP levels, which could mean a lot of different things. A big one is spina bifida, which is a spine disorder that can be fixed with simple surgery, or it can lead to water in the brain and a bunch of terminal issues.

And the thing about this whole process is that it produces thoughts that make you question your own morals. Heidi and I would never terminate a pregnancy, but in the moment, you can't help but wonder, *If the baby will be burdened with all these major issues, would it be better if she didn't make it at all?* Even just thinking about that makes you feel like a horrible person, but you can't help all those thoughts swirling inside your head.

A doctor then called us into the ultrasound room, and we sat down. My whole body tightened as I reached over and held Heidi's hand. The doctor turned off the light and flipped on the ultrasound machine. As the machine whirred to life, it shone onto a giant projection screen on the wall, and a split second later, a crystal-clear image of our baby filled the screen.

And in that instant, all my fears vanished.

Looking at our child, I couldn't see anything other than perfection. I didn't care about all the hardships that might come down the road. All I saw was our kid, our baby, and nothing else mattered. In that moment, she was perfect to me no matter what.

For ten minutes, we marveled at our baby as the doctor examined her. Then she turned to us and told us that everything was fine. The baby was the perfect size and the perfect length, and there were no issues at all. And then the doctor was nice enough to give us an envelope that revealed the gender of our baby.

We were presented with a question: *Do we open the envelope or not?* If we did open it, would we want to make an announcement? Who would we tell?

But we would decide that later. We were just celebrating our healthy baby (Juniper).

Things She'll Say During the **Second** Trimester

"Babe, you know what I want to do? So you wanna?"

"I can't get pregnant again. This is like a freebie. You don't want a freebie?"

"My skin looks so good. My nails look so good. My hair looks so good."

"Look at all these new curves I got. I could be in a rap video."

"Mama's got energy back. It's time to work out."

(Five minutes later) "That's a good workout. I really hit hard today. I need a nap."

"I'm going to finish making this baby in six months. How long is it going to take you to finish fixing up the house?"

"Babe, my butt is more pregnant than my belly."

"Hey, while you're up, can you get the pickles and the ice cream and the jelly and the cashews? Shut up. Just put it in a bowl and bring it over here. You did this."

"I peed myself seven times today. What did *you* do?"

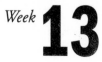

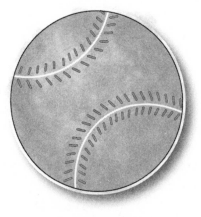

BASEBALL

Your little dude's got his organs in place and his muscles and nerves have formed, and he is currently the size of a baseball. That means he's now stretching and flexing his arms and legs like a baseball player might do while waiting for his next at bat. But it's gonna be a while before your slugger can hit a dinger. He's just hanging out in his dugout (aka the amniotic sac), and he has lots of room to do some squats or scratch his groin. Well, he doesn't exactly have one—not yet.

The baby's coach, Mommy, doesn't feel any movements right now. But hopefully it'll be a whole new ball game as those first-trimester issues like morning sickness and fatigue start to subside. The achy, irritated, and exhausted feelings will still be there, just like the kind you feel when you decide to eat four chili dogs at the ballpark.

Baseball was a big part of my childhood. Every summer was spent traveling to small towns all over South Dakota to play Little League.

The first few years I played, my dad was the coach, which was fun but also meant I batted first. He coached my team simply because no other dads volunteered to do it. But the reality was, my dad didn't know squat about baseball. He also was a traveling salesman, which in South Dakota meant he drove a lot, and his territory covered most of the eastern half of the state. But all summer long, at least once or twice a week, he would rearrange his schedule to drive two or three hours back to whatever little town we were playing in.

A few years went by, I joined a new team with a new coach, and my dad was now off the hook from coaching. I went from batting first to batting last in one year. This could have been because my dad was no longer coaching. But it also might have been because all my teammates hit puberty and grew a head taller than me. I'd like to think I was a pretty decent ballplayer, but I definitely lost my edge when I became the smallest kid on the team. It didn't matter, though; even though he was no longer coaching, my dad was still at every game.

To me the moral of the story is this: It doesn't matter if your kid bats first or last.

What matters is that you're at the game.

DAD DUTY

So you just read this and shrugged, thinking, *Well, that's nice. I'll make sure I'm there for my kid's games, but that's down the road.*

Yeah, but you know what's also down the road? Your wife's obstetrician. And you know what you can do? Go to the appointment with her.

Whether you think you need to be there or not, go with her. She wants you to be there, so just go. Don't ask her whether or not you should. Just ask her the date and time of the appointment.

If it's your third pregnancy and you have two other kiddos to deal with, then maybe you don't have to go to *all* the appointments—just a couple of the big ones. But if it's your first baby, GO!

Here's a conversation between an oblivious guy and his pregnant wife.

"Are you going to come to my first doctor's appointment?" pregnant wife asks.

"I don't know," oblivious guy replies. "What would I be there for?"

She's not asking whether or not you want to go. This is her way of saying you'd better freaking come.

Just go. Be with her. Ask questions. Be involved. Learn something.

You'll never regret it.

BABIES VERSUS ADULTS (FIRST WEEK WITH BABY)

Your first week with your baby is going to be monumental. You'll experience lots of things that week. Here's the first discovery I made about newborns: They're exactly like that one terrible friend in college that calls you up in the middle of the night and wants to go out and paint the town red. So you're like, "Okay, I better go out with you just to babysit you." He ends up drinking the entire bottle, getting super dramatic, pooping himself, and then passing out in your bed. Yep, pretty similar.

There are a lot of amazing things about newborns—way more amazing, in fact, than similar things in us grown-ups.

The first thing about newborns: Their sneezes are adorable. They could end wars. Adults' sneezes, not so much. Those can sound like either a hyena's cry or a car backfiring.

Another awesome thing about babies is they have zero control over their limbs. Their limbs look like the arms of the inflatable tube man. This would suck as an adult. Especially as someone who enjoys hot coffee.

Babies pass out in the middle of a meal. Just nursing and guzzling and then zzzing and dreaming. Again, this would suck as an adult. Especially if you enjoy hot soup.

Another awesome thing about babies is how swinging them and giving them a pacifier completely chills them out. Okay, this would be awesome if it worked on adults. Imagine that frantic day with phone calls and meetings and emails and voicemails and stress and drama and then—boom. Binky in the mouth. Body in the swing . . . There would be swing sets in every office building.

Pure bliss.

Babies smell amazing. That new-baby smell is better than pine trees. You bury your nose in his neck and inhale the sweet scent of his skin. Now imagine doing that to your co-worker Frank. Probably not the best idea. That might lead to an interesting conversation with HR.

It's crazy how well babies sleep. Adults, not so much. We sleep around a baby's schedule. Well, we try to. We know we should sleep when she sleeps, but when the house is finally quiet, we just want to chill out and have some time to ourselves. Maybe binge-watch old episodes of *The Office*. Then when we finally go to bed—WAAAHHHH! Baby's up.

Enjoy that first week. Like shaving for the first time, you'll get to do it only once.

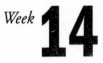
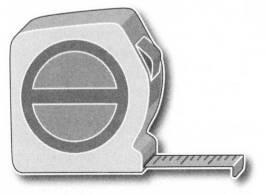

TAPE MEASURE

For week 14, let's assess how baby and Mommy are doing right now.

Baby: Let's measure the baby. Actually, he's right around the size of a tape measure! These come in lots of sizes, but think of your classic tape measure with twenty-five feet of tape. Since every baby is growing at a slightly different pace, let's give or take a centimeter or two.

Something else starting to grow is the hair on your little tape measure. Babies grow body hair called lanugo. It's like a cozy blanket that keeps them warm. They'll shed this before being born, unless they're related to Chewbacca.

Also, consider this crazy fact: A boy begins to develop a prostate gland around now, and a girl's ovaries are beginning to shift down into her pelvis.

Mommy: Hopefully your lady is starting to feel more peppy and less pukey. Those first-trimester symptoms begin to settle down, and those trips to the bathroom get less frequent. She might be feeling a little more comfortable in her own body. *So you wanna . . . ?* And chances are she's gonna start wanting to too.

THE MARKINGS OF A GOOD PARENT

So why do we use a tape measure for our projects? We use it because it shows us the same measurements, no matter where we take it. It's the exact same every time you pull it out; the markings remain unchanged. There is consistency. In the same way, we're meant to be a constant in the lives of our children. Three feet, four inches *always* needs to be three feet, four inches. I'm not saying this is *easy*, but I am saying it's important.

Early on, your job as a father will basically be to keep your child alive. But when she becomes a toddler, you and your wife will become fluent in the language of "No." Disciplining a child is ridiculously challenging because you're constantly walking this line between *I don't want to be a pushover* and *I feel like I yell all day long*. At first I felt like my disciplining was sort of all over the place—yelling, screaming, time-out, time-in, occasionally just looking the other way. I finally realized I couldn't just wing it and get it right. So I purchased a couple of books and did a little reading (just like you're doing right now—kudos to you). This is what I learned.

One definition of *discipline* is actually "to teach"; it's not "to punish." Instead of yelling, "Hey! Don't throw your balls in the bush, or you're going to get a time-out!" I explain, "Don't throw your balls in the bush, or your balls will be in the bush, and you won't have any more balls." You can also redirect your kid. In the toddler stage, your kiddo is becoming an individual with all his own desires and curiosity, which he exhibits through lots of exploration. It's difficult for kids to live inside our dull adult parameters, where you can't just put anything you want in the toilet (how lame is that?). While it's sometimes very necessary to reprimand them, at other times it's much more effective to redirect them. Not only are you accomplishing your goal, but you're also teaching your kid something new that he might want to do more.

I've had to also learn to tone it down. It's tough to moderate your own reaction when your kid is putting your TV remote in the toilet. But if you come in with big emotion, your child will likely react with big emotion. If you throw a tantrum, your child is also going to throw a tantrum. One of us has to be the adult. Sometimes I can't help wondering, *Why does it always have to be me?*

One of the traps I often get into is expecting our kids to follow the rules today because they followed them yesterday. But toddlers' minds are still developing. That's why you're going to need to not only explain the rules but also kindly and lovingly enforce them over and over again before they get it. You gotta be like that tape measure—consistent in your responses to their behaviors.

Even though your baby is the size of a tape measure right around now, one day your child is going to view you as a tape measure—the constant, steady one. We're what our kids are using to understand and evaluate life. We have to be consistent in setting good examples for them, making good boundaries, and remaining steady and true. Life is way harder when there is no consistency for your kid, when your parenting looks more like a Magic 8 Ball than a tape measure. One of the things that makes this so challenging is that we as dads have to be constant when everything around us is changing. I know it's not easy, fellas, but you got this!

When you're disciplining, ask yourself the following question: *Am I doing this because I'm mad at them, or am I doing it because I love them?* Because, at the end of the day, our goal should be to help our kids. It's to teach them, guide them, and mold them into responsible, kind adults that do the right thing not because they're told to but because they want to. Discipline is just as much about us as it is about them. For the most part, we don't know what we're doing. And that's okay—we're all learning as we go. Just like our kids need to hear the same things over and over again, we need to do the same things over and over again so that our expectations become predictable. That way our measurements stay the same, time and time again. Measure twice and cut once, my friend.

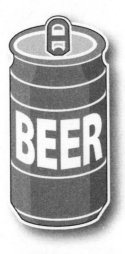

BEER CAN

Pull up a chair. Here's a beer. Let's talk man to man. Dude to dude. Dad to dad.

Now look at that twelve-ounce can you're holding; that's about the size of your little one right now. Go ahead—hold it up to your chest and rock it. Cuddle it. Tell it how excited you are to be its dad. Just don't open it for a minute now, or it will spray everywhere.

So let me help you dial it in with even more detail since I'm clearly the expert here. Behold: Your baby's eyes. He has eyebrows and eyelids and eyelashes. What color do you think his eyes will be one day? Now look at his fingers and toes. They have nails. Watch him for a moment. Yep, that's right. He's yawning and stretching and wiggling his toes. Wait—look there! He's sucking his thumb!

Don't worry, Dad. Mom won't be able to feel all this. Not yet.

If you could take an X-ray, it would show your baby's bones, which are starting to harden. By now your baby's spinal cord is completely formed.

Now it's time to set down the beer and switch topics. What? You finished it already? You rascal! Okay, so your wife is now in her second trimester, which means she's less nauseous and fatigued and might start feeling more "frisky" than ever. I'll let you do the math . . . but one suggestion I have for you is that it might be a great time to start thinking about how you're presenting yourself.

It's time for a man makeover.

MAN MAKEOVER

Let's face it, guys—we aren't always the best at taking care of ourselves. We get married, we get comfortable, and we stop trying as hard. We drink too many craft IPAs and inevitably build an awning over our "tools." Let me tell you now—after you have kids, fitness will become ten times harder. So start thinking about it now. What changes can you make to not only look healthier but also feel healthier? Can you cut down on your pizza intake? Eat more veggies? What's your exercise regimen look like? Are you paying attention to your mental and emotional health? Have you changed your style since 2005? Are you thinking about any of this, or are you slowly letting yourself go?

Before you start taking care of someone else, you need to make sure you're taking care of yourself. The healthier you are, the better equipped you will be. Kids take an enormous amount of physical, mental, and emotional energy. Your kids are also going to look at you as an example of how to live. You need to become the man you want your sons to be and the man you want your daughters to marry. It's like those oxygen masks on the plane. You gotta put yours on first. Talk with your partner about how you can structure your new life to make sure you each have the me time that makes you feel whole. Find a friend who is in the same stage of life. Buy a really good book that will give you enormous amounts of fantastic advice (boom—nailed it).

This is all big-picture lifestyle stuff, but if you want some quick and easy "help me look sexier to my wife" advice, here you go. Get a fitted T-shirt. Stop wearing the same old baggy hardware-store T-shirt, and get something that's made for your body type. Wear hats less, get a professional haircut, and learn how to style your hair. If you don't have hair, that's okay. Mr. Clean is bald, and women think he's basically the sexiest man alive. Then again . . . maybe that's because he cleans a lot. Maybe *you* should clean a lot. At the end of the day, just ask your wife. Let her dress you. If she thinks you look good, that's all that matters. Make a date of it. Go to the mall, and let her pick out your clothes. Sure, you might end up with some questionable shirts from Nordstrom Rack, but you also might get lucky (and I don't mean the jeans).

LESSON TO MODEL FOR YOUR KID

Beer is something to enjoy after a hard day's work, not a reason to not go into work. Same goes for *Fortnite*.

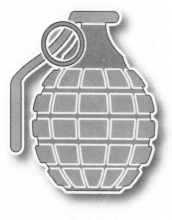

GRENADE

High five, little guy—you're now as big as a grenade. Dad, if you, like me, have never actually held a grenade before, then let's say it's about the size of your closed fist. Little monster *is* mounting a clear offensive, and your lady might start to feel some movement in her abdomen. Some people call it flutters; I call it freaking marine baby boot camp. Baby isn't fluttering; he's working out—bicycle kicks and umbilical cord rope climbs. It's like a little CrossFit gym in there. Also like a marine, he's collecting intelligence. He can now hear your voice and will develop the capacity to recognize it upon birth. Now would be a good time to start reciting every line from *Die Hard* to your wife's stomach. "Welcome to the party, pal." Just walk past your wife and yell "Hans!" She'll love it. Your baby will get to know your voice and be thoroughly entertained. Your wife may be indifferent. It's tragic, but a lot of wives don't fully appreciate the Willis.

"COME OUT TO THE COAST. WE'LL GET TOGETHER, HAVE A FEW LAUGHS . . ."

Soon your baby will burst out and blast your life with sleepless nights and smelly diapers and unconditional love, but you have a brief time before the weapon detonates. Discovering you're pregnant is like being handed a live grenade; the months leading up to the birth are those four seconds before it blows up. And that explosion is going to change your life in the best way.

Your friends who haven't decided to start breeding won't understand. How can they? It's not really their fault. While you're setting up the new crib, they're backpacking across Europe. Suddenly you don't see them anymore. You won't be going out for beers or playing golf or doing any of that fun stuff, since it's very difficult to do that with a kid in tow. Have you ever tried to golf eighteen holes while wearing an infant in a BabyBjörn? I've done it and it's not easy. My handicap went up like twenty strokes. You *will* do fun stuff—just not nearly as much. The only way friends will get to hang out with you is if they come to your house; you can't go to their house, because your kid will break their stuff. And it's honestly best if they come kick it after your kiddo goes to bed.

You know how they say kids say the darndest things? Well, so do friends without kids. Here's a list of ridiculous things my friends without kids have said to me:

"I don't have kids, but my dog . . ."
No, your Yorkie-poo is not like our baby. Not even close. Even if you do put tiny sweaters on him.

"Ah man, I'm so busy right now. No, Friday is no good. That's my poker night."
Oh, you're so busy? Taking care of . . . you? Must be tough.

"I think I slept too much last night. Now I'm just exhausted."
Poor you. I'm sorry for your loss.

"What do you mean you're not going to be there? Just get a babysitter."

As much as I want to go out every chance I get, babysitters add up. Also, just finding a babysitter that you actually trust can suck.

"You don't have any time for your friends anymore."

It's not that I don't have time for you. It's that I don't have time . . . at all. The other night, I spent forty-five minutes trying to convince my son to eat pizza. Not broccoli—pizza. Also, I brush another person's teeth.

The reality is your friend group is going to go through some changes. Your die-hard friends without kids will stick with you and adjust as needed. Others will have kids at the same time, and these folks will naturally understand what you're going through. The shared life experience is going to make them some of your closest friends. And there are some that you'll just stop hanging out with. It's not on purpose, it's not personal, but you'll lose touch. Very naturally you'll find out which of your friends are going to be a big part of this next chapter of your life. You're going to find out which friends are willing to jump on the grenade with you.

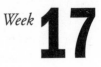

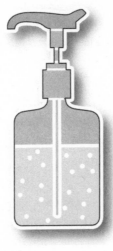

BOTTLE OF SANITIZER

Your little bottle of joy is now the size of a fourteen-ounce bottle of hand sanitizer.

Don't you love it when you squirt some sanitizer onto your hand and suddenly it's covered in thick, gooey, dripping sauce that smells like a leftover shot of tequila stuck in your trash can? We're all aware by now that not all sanitizer is created equal, and coming off a worldwide pandemic, we know more about sanitizer than we ever thought we would.

Speaking of gooey sauce, did you know that your baby is now smothered with a slimy white substance that protects her skin from the amniotic fluid surrounding her? This is called vernix caseosa, but you can just think of it as your baby being dipped in fresh queso. That's way better than knockoff hand sanitizer, am I right?

A LITTLE DIRT DON'T HURT

A lot of parents get freaked out about their kids getting dirty, but I for one have never been scared of a little dirt. However, after becoming a father and seeing how incredibly dirty my kids can get in almost no time, I decided it was a good idea to do some research. This is what I found.

We're living in the era of sterilization. Parents are practically bathing their children in hand sanitizer, and kids are spending just half as much time outside as twenty years ago when I was growing up. So you would think the kids living in this cleaner environment would be healthier, but it's actually the exact opposite. There are way more allergies and asthma today. And here's the kicker. Researchers are saying it's *because of the clean environment*! Who knew?

Let me break it down for you. A baby's immune system is a lot like a baby's brain. That brain needs stimulation, interaction, and input to help it develop. In that sense, preventing a dog from licking your baby's face is essentially like not reading a book to him. You're denying his body the chance to interact with microscopic organisms that can be essential to the development of his immune system.

That's a mouthful.

"Microscopic organisms?" you ask. "You mean germs, right?"

Let me break it down further. Microscopic organisms, also known as microbes, are literally everywhere. Some good, some bad. Which microbes are good? Soil-based organisms. That's right . . . *dirt.*

I know what you might be thinking.

All right, Taylor. Sounds like you're using a lot of ten-dollar words to say that dirt is good. Can you just give me a specific example?

Absolutely. So when babies are first born, all they eat is milk, and breast milk has hardly any iron, which is good because pathogens like *E. coli* thrive on iron and can cause severe digestive problems in newborns. Once babies are about six months old, they need more iron in their diet, but they're not getting any from the milk. Luckily, that's also the exact same time that they start crawling around and getting in the dirt. And what's great about dirt? It's a great source of iron. It's almost like it was designed that way. (I don't know if you can tell, but I really love this stuff!)

Don't just take it from me; go do your own research. I've realized that, to do the right thing in this particular situation, we just have to do less. Kids already want to play in the dirt. All we have to do is not freak out, which is awesome because that's what I was already doing. See—this parenting stuff isn't so hard!

FIVE PEOPLE WHO VISIT
THE NEW BABY

1. The Baby Hog (aka Grandma)

"Where's that baby? Gimme, gimme, gimme."

"Oh, I see you, son. You're chopped liver. Where's the baby?"

"Now, I know you said you had enough blankets, but I crocheted these on the way."

"Grandma's got him. Grandma's got him. NOBODY TOUCH HIM—GRANDMA'S GOT IT!"

2. The Nervous Nellie

"Cute kid . . . Oh no, I don't need to hold her."

"Oh, it's okay. Let somebody else have a turn."

"What's that? I have to do what? Why do I have to support his head? What's wrong with his head?"

"Oh no, is she breathing? She's not doing anything."

"No, I'm not standing up. I'll drop her."

"Somebody please take him. Take him, take him, take him, take him!"

3. The Know-It-All

"Oh, sweetie . . . Can I give you some advice?"

"Why are you swaddling her so tight? You got her wrapped up like one of them Chipotle burritos."

"Oh no, I'm sorry. I just thought you wanted your kids to be healthy."

"I breastfed all three of my boys. Now one of them's an engineer. *Structural.*"

"No, he ain't latching. Let me help you out there. Let me get in there. He doesn't have a good latch. Not just a little tip like that—he needs the whole teat."

"I'm not a doctor, but . . ."

"Is that your pediatrician? Let me talk to him. Give me the phone."

4. Mr. Oblivious

"Oh, whatcha got here? A neck pillow? Oh, that feels pretty good!"

"What's that sour smell?"

"Paternity leave? We ain't having none of that. Dory was at home with all four kids right after the birth, and I was straight back to the office. You were fine, weren't you, Dory? What's that look?"

"Oh, just going to breastfeed right out here? I'm gonna go fix the garage door."

"Hey, son, you got to do something about your wife. She just flashed me."

5. The Drop-and-Run

"Oh, sorry. We didn't want to bother you. You've got enough on your plate; you don't need us in there. We'll come back another time once you've settled in, okay?"

"Oh, the baby is sleeping, so we shouldn't come in."

"No, really, you need your rest. We can't stay. Gotta go."

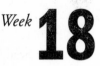
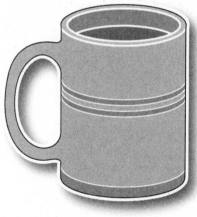

CUP OF COFFEE

It's morning. Time to grind those coffee beans to make your wife a cappuccino that you can serve her in one of the forty-two mugs she's impulse bought . . . LIVE LAUGH COFFEE. But check with her first because she might not be drinking as much caffeine these days. Maybe a decaf cappuccino will do the trick.

Your baby is now the same size as the cup of coffee. The tiny bones in your baby's ears have started to harden, and the nerves from her brain are connected to her ears, meaning she can hear the grinder pulverizing those beans. Curled up, she's probably almost six inches long, and she weighs around seven ounces, a lot less than that Venti salted caramel mocha Frappuccino you just picked up in the drive-through at Starbucks.

Hopefully you bought a drink for your wife. She surely needs a pick-me-up since she's feeling so loaded down. Literally. That expanding baby causes her center of gravity to shift forward, placing stress on her spine and producing some major back pain. She's also feeling more light-headed because the increase in progesterone is making her blood vessels relax. That means more blood going to the baby but less blood coming back to Mommy, causing her to feel dizzy.

Something else that might be low is her blood sugar. Maybe you should just give your Frappuccino to your wife. And also grab a jar of pickles . . . She might want those too.

IF YOU BREW IT, THEY WILL COME

Coffee. I love coffee. I've made the bad habit of drinking it every day. I've made the even-worse habit of buying it every day. I'm not sure why, but there is always part of me that would rather pay five bucks for someone else to make it than make the exact same thing at home. Sure, I know how to make my own coffee, but somehow it tastes better if somebody else makes it. Maybe it's because it's one less thing I have to worry about or because it feels like I'm treating myself. *The kids were insane at school drop-off today, so I've earned this.* Regardless of why, I just assume that this other person can make the coffee better because that's her job. She has all the fancy equipment, and I give her the benefit of the doubt.

Here's the reality: That barista who's making your drink might be a seventeen-year-old kid on her third day at the job, so she might not know better than you. If you drink your coffee every day, you know how it's supposed to taste, but we give the barista the benefit of the doubt that she's doing it right. When I'm doing it myself, I honestly don't really know if I'm making the shots with the right consistency or if the froth is Starbucks-worthy. When somebody else is doing it, however, I'm like, *Cool, she's got it.*

Parenting can feel a lot like this. Around other parents, it's easy to get self-conscious about whether we're doing it right. But nobody really knows if they're doing it right. It just seems like the other parents know how to do things better, because we ourselves feel completely lost. So how can you know for sure? It's your child, so shouldn't you, the parent, know best? Not always . . .

I hate it when people say, "Parents know best." While in some cases that is most definitely true, in others it couldn't be further from the truth. Just because someone procreated doesn't mean that he now has infinite knowledge about parenting. It really comes down to how much time and effort he's putting into understanding how to effectively communicate with and parent each of his children.

What I've learned about parenting is that I should always try multiple approaches. If you always do what you've always done, you'll always get what you've always got. It's like experimenting with how to make coffee—sometimes you have to try different things in order to get the best cup of joe you can. We recently purchased our own espresso machine in order to save some money (we'll see how that goes). So I've learned the basics of steaming milk and pulling shots. My drinks taste okay, but the shots definitely aren't as strong. I could just keep making them the exact same way and be okay with mediocre lattes, or I could dive deeper and learn more about my specific machine as well as the beans I'm using. How coarse should my grind be? How much should I pack the grind? How hot should I steam the milk? How much foam?

Why not think in these terms when it comes to our kids? As a father, you need to be willing to ask for help from someone you might be able to learn from. Read books, watch videos, and talk with your dad friends. At the end of the day, you *will* be the expert on your own kid—but only if you're actually putting in the work. There is a balance here, a place in the middle. You're going to have to give yourself some credit and stop thinking that every other parent out there knows more than you. But you also have to check yourself to make sure that you deserve the credit. That you're doing the best job you can be doing. You'll need coffee, I assure you. Fatherhood is exhausting. But if you're exhausted, it means only one thing—*you're doing it right.*

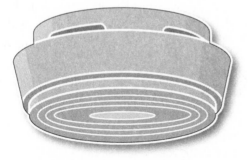

FIRE ALARM

Do you hear that? A fire alarm is going off! But this is one fire you don't want to stop. These are flames of celebration. IT'S GENDER REVEAL TIME, BABY!

Before you can actually pull off a gender reveal, you have to know if that little bun in the oven is a boy or a girl. And around this time, between weeks 18 and 20, moms will get another ultrasound scan that thoroughly checks the baby's structural development. By now the baby is almost fully formed, with organs functioning at an advanced level. Eyes remain closed until around week 26, but they're in their final position just like the ears. Even a baby's fingerprints are starting to form.

Let's say you decide to find out the gender. This is where you might venture into the controversial territory of gender reveals. For one of our gender reveals, we did a Rube Goldberg machine video that went viral, and with that came lots of love and support as well as some oddly Negative Nancies. And I get it. Yes, there are people out there that have gone too far, and yes, there are some people that hate their lives. So let's get this out of the way . . . These are the things *not* to do during a gender reveal:

1. Do NOT shoot unstabilized fireworks that tip over and launch at your family and friends.
2. Do NOT start a fire that burns forty-five thousand acres of a national forest.
3. Do NOT strike your wife with a bat after swinging at the baseball filled with powder. And don't blast your wife with said powder.
4. Do NOT crash the plane that you're using to dump out 350 gallons of pink water for the big reveal.
5. Do NOT shoot yourself in the groin with the confetti cannon during the big moment.
6. Do NOT shoot your brother in the groin with the confetti cannon during the big moment.
7. Do NOT create a pipe bomb that accidentally kills the family dog.

All these are actual events that have happened. Yes, people make mistakes, and sometimes parents can simply be irresponsible. So be smart. The thing to remember when doing anything big and dangerous is *ready, aim, fire*. It's not *ready, fire, aim*. If you keep that process in the right order, you'll decrease your chances of turning your celebration into an "incident." It's not good to go viral for the wrong reasons.

But don't let all the Negative Nancies and naysayers taint your excitement. As far as I'm concerned, I haven't gone too far. I haven't gone far enough! This is huge and exciting and life changing.

As for the Debbie Downers, don't tell me I can't be excited about this! This baby is going to be a part of the rest of my life. I currently know almost *nothing* about my kid, but I'm about to find out the genitals, and by golly, I want to celebrate! Get out of my way, internet police! This is our baby; we're going to celebrate! If you want to celebrate, too, then watch the damn video! If you don't—*whoosh*—swipe up, ya BITTY!

Sorry about that. But seriously, if we get pregnant again, I'm renting Elon Musk's Tesla Cannon and blasting off into orbit when we do the gender reveal. That's how exciting it should feel to you. It's like this is *your* birthday party and you're about to unwrap the presents, and *oh my freaking goodness, this is the best day ever!* How pumped are you right now, bro, 'cause this is awesome! If you want to have a gender reveal party, then have a gender reveal party! If you don't, cool. You do you.

I've listed the things *not* to do, so here are a few things to think about:

1. Who do you tell? Is it an intimate moment between husband and wife, or are you going to make a live pay-per-view event on social media? Make sure you select a time and a place and then let those people know.
2. What theme will you pick? There are thousands of ideas online. Think about your professions and hobbies. Do you want to do something physical like popping balloons, or would you rather it be some sort of presentation like revving your dirt bike?
3. Is it dangerous? And if so, is it something you've done before? Make sure you're confident about safely performing the feat, whether it's skydiving or launching some sort of missile or simply swinging at a piñata.
4. Do you have a backup plan for an emergency?
5. Do you have health insurance and life insurance?
6. Do you live near dry, grassy fields or an oil refinery?
7. Is your wife even comfortable around sharks?

Okay, well, these are just a few things to get your brain asking important questions.

Of course, there is also the flip side of couples that don't want to find out the gender. The "we'll just wait" parents. That's fine too. We wanted to wait to learn the gender of our first baby, but then during our last doctor's visit one week before Theo was born, he accidentally showed us the testicles. And I was like, "Ah nuts!"

Testicles? WHAT? It's a boy! *Yep, those are testicles, so that means we're going to jump bikes together and build fires and go snowboarding and go wakeboarding. Or maybe he won't be into any of that and I'll learn a new hobby. Either way, we're having a boy and it's going to be awesome.*

Last bit of advice: If you don't want to find out the gender of your baby, tell your doctor. And tell the nurse and the PA and the medical assistant and literally everyone waiting in the lobby that you're *waitin' to find out.* And do this every time you make a doctor's visit.

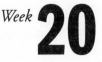

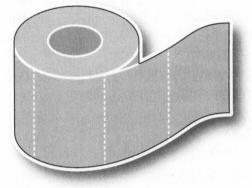

FRESH ROLL OF TOILET PAPER

Let's talk about pee-pee and doo-doo. Number one and number two. Tinkle and poopy-doops.

Laugh all you want . . . One day, with a completely straight face, you'll be using similar terms when talking about the bathroom with your child.

Right around now, your baby is the size of a fresh roll of toilet paper, and his digestive system is starting to function. He's guzzling amniotic fluid now, meaning that whatever Mommy eats, he'll be tasting as well. The Cheesy Gordita Crunch your wife couldn't help ordering? *Sabe bueno!* The zesty dill pickles and Oreo ice cream combo? Bring it on! Gouda pizza smothered with sauerkraut? Why not!

DADS AND DIAPERS

The days when you'll wipe only your own tush are coming to a close, my friend. Pretty soon you'll be helping change diapers. Wait . . . Did you think that was just Mom's responsibility? Oh boy, you might need to adjust your expectations just a tad.

Here's the thing. Diapers don't start out weighing ten pounds and dripping all over your new carpet. Just like many things with parenting, you get to ease into the whole diaper business.

After your baby is born, she'll have very simple needs. She's either hungry, tired, bored, or lonely. Parents are there to meet those basic needs, like feeding her or shushing her. Things start out simple. It can feel intense because your baby needs something nearly all the time, but the range of what she needs is relatively limited. Every time you hear a cry, it's almost like a multiple choice question. If you don't get it right with (A) hungry, try (B) poopy diaper. If it's not (B) poopy diaper, try (C) tired. Over time your child will become more and more complex, as will her problems and needs. One day you're no longer worried about her physical needs. She can feed herself. She can change herself. But now you have to walk her through her best friend calling her a "cottonheaded ninnymuggins" or her crush breaking her heart. As her life becomes more complex, so do her needs.

Diapers are kind of the same way. Newborns are pretty much consuming only milk, so all that comes out is this yellow poopy resembling mustard. It doesn't have too much odor, and those diapers are super easy to change. As they eat more and more solids, things get more intense. The good news is that you don't have to deal with that right away. Think about it like a *Super Mario Bros.* game. You don't instantly have to worry about beating the big enemy, Wario. At first all you have to worry about is jumping on mushroom heads. Things get harder as you level up. So don't be scared of diapers, because you're going to get lots of practice on the easy ones before you have to face a total Bowser blowout.

THAT'S A SPICY MEATBALL!

Speaking of food, when was the last time you made a meal for your lady? This week, why don't you surprise her one night by making dinner?

No, that doesn't mean picking up some lasagna at Olive Garden or swinging by Chili's for some Chicken Crispers. I'm talking about going into the kitchen and creating an actual meal that requires a recipe and ingredients.

Don't have a recipe book? I'm sure you do. Look again. Check in the upper cabinets. If you find baking supplies, you're probably close. If you can't find it, you can use one of the sixteen million recipes they have online.

Think about some of *her* favorite foods. Don't just make sloppy joes because that's what you're craving. After all, she's carrying your offspring—literally growing a human! Use this as an opportunity to thoughtfully express your appreciation. Maybe even make some side dishes (Cool Ranch Doritos are not a side dish).

Don't forget to clean up. If the kitchen looks like a high school science lab, she's going to lose her appetite, and you're going to be up sh** creek without a paddle.

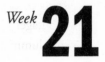

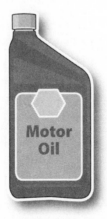

QUART OF OIL

The worst part about a car breaking down is when you're out on the road [and] you're a guy. Because now you have to get out and pretend like you know what you're doing . . . You're looking in there [under the hood]. You know, you're hoping you're going to see something in there so simple, so obvious, so incredibly easy to fix, even you can handle it. Like a giant on/off switch turned off.

—JERRY SEINFELD

Guys have to fix things, don't we? Even if we have no idea how to fix something, we still have to go through the motions of trying to figure out what's wrong. It's a man thing. We want to use every one of those 3,479 tools we *definitely* need in our garage, even though we really use only like twelve of them. Nobody wants to act like they don't have a clue.

Plumbing issue? *Let me check the pipes.*

Power outage? *Let me check the breakers.*

Meteor plummeting to the earth? *Let me take a look at 'er!*

A lot of guys are doers. We like to be fixers. We like to take charge. I think that's why pregnancy can be difficult for us. There's nothing for us to fix. Sure, we can help out around the house and support and humor our wives, but we can't do anything to fix the morning sickness or the aching back. Sure, we can go out and get that food she's craving or help support that pillow behind her back, but we can't really fix anything in the fullest sense. And what's there to fix? Pregnancy is a beautiful and mysterious and amazing thing that a woman experiences in her own body. We're along for the ride for sure, but we're in the passenger seat. So when the car breaks down, all we can do is be patient and hold the flashlight.

One thing we can do, though, is check the oil. Oil lubricates the car's engine and keeps it running smoothly. This is where we fit in during pregnancy. We can do whatever it takes to help our wives keep running. Here are some things you can do to keep the engine firing on all cylinders:

1. Make time for a walk together every morning. This will help her stay active, but it will also give you time to check in with each other.
2. Become her personal chef and caterer. Starbucks run? Check. Taco Tuesday night? You got it handled. She's craving cucumber and ham on rye bread with ranch dressing? Make a run to the grocery store.
3. Do the house chores. Instead of taking the dirty clothes basket to the laundry room, why not just go ahead and do the laundry? Don't just put some dishes in the dishwasher— program the cycles, and then take the clean dishes out. Make the bed. Scrub the shower. Clean your bathroom counter. Clean all the things that you don't normally clean.

4. Declutter. No, I'm not talking about the decorative items around the house. Can you clean the garage? How about going through the storage and loading up the car with things for Goodwill? You'll soon be filling that garage and storage area with lots of baby-related stuff.

5. Read some books on pregnancy and parenting (check out the bibliography in the back of the book for some recommendations). This is a great place to start if you're trying to figure out where to pitch in. Use what you've read as conversation starters with your lady. I guarantee she's already thinking about whatever you might bring up. Or invite her to read this book with you. It's totally wife friendly. Heidi made sure.

6. Help her with her monthly belly pics. This may seem strange to you, but they're amazing keepsakes for her since they document the journey her body went through.

7. Here's the simplest, most important thing—listen to your wife.

Don't try to fix everything. Just listen. Be patient. Make eye contact, and try to begin to fathom what she's going through. Don't give advice; give your wife the opportunity to simply ask for it if she wants to.

Try this challenge: Come up with a personalized list of engine maintenance ideas that you know will help your lady.

Speaking of engine maintenance, your baby is now the size of a quart of oil. Did you know his brain is starting to develop nerve pathways that communicate details like temperature and pressure and pain? It will be quite a few weeks before his brain will recognize these signals. But now his movements are more coordinated instead of twitchy and jerky because the cartilage in his body is turning into bone.

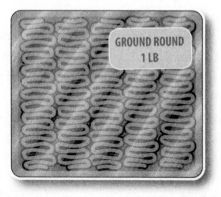

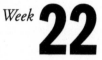

POUND OF GROUND BEEF

Your baby is now approximately the same weight as that pack of frozen ground beef you buy at the grocery store. Baby is developing the senses she'll one day use to hear and see and smell that delicious sizzling meat you make into a scrumptious meal. Her hands are in constant motion as well, practicing for the day they snatch something off the stovetop when you've looked away.

Ground beef is a key ingredient in a lot of dishes. It's versatile. It's like the Swiss Army Knife of meats. You can make chili or spaghetti with it. You can make a shepherd's pie or a patty melt. The recipes are endless—beef and bean burritos, taco salad, stuffed peppers, slow-cooker hamburger hash, and on and on. But I'd be willing to wager that two dishes reign supreme in the realm of most often cooked.

Hamburgers and tacos.

Most people stop at those common and unoriginal recipes.

Similarly, it's easy to fall into a routine during pregnancy. Remember, you're already past the halfway mark, and it's easy to become complacent or feel as if you're not able to contribute much.

Come on, gentlemen. Don't succumb to that reductionistic way of thinking. You have so much to offer, and it might be time to add some new dishes to your repertoire.

DEFROSTING

Right now it probably feels like all you're doing is waiting for your baby and watching your wife from the sidelines. But you really have two options at this juncture. You can just sit on your butt while the ground beef thaws, or you can start fixing onion to add to it. You can prepare some sides. You can set out the condiments. You can clean up the kitchen even before all the cooking is done. You can fix your wife a Shirley Temple.

Guys have nine months to prepare to become a father. Consider this time a great opportunity to plan ahead and plot out the course your family will take once your baby is born. Sure, you don't know all the details, but you can do so many things while standing by. Start thinking about what kind of father you want to be. Do you want to be just like your dad? Or maybe there are a few things you'd like to do differently? What are the most important things you want to teach your kid? What kinds of adventures do you want to have as a family? How do you want to handle sleep training and discipline? How do you want to discuss sports and school and big questions about God? Now is a good time to have some conversations with your lady about these things so that you have the same game plan. You might not align on every topic, but the sooner you start talking about your family culture, the more likely you are to have a unified vision when baby arrives.

I'm a big believer in dreaming big and watching your dreams come true. Dream about what kind of family you want to have. Dream about what kind of dad you want to be. And most importantly, start preparing to see those dreams become a reality, my friend. This is going to be the best ground beef of your life.

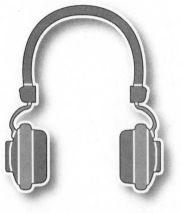

BOSE NOISE-CANCELING
HEADPHONES

Come on—feel the noise!

Around now your baby's personal recording booth starts to lose its soundproof insulation, meaning he can now hear a dog barking or Quiet Riot playing (which may actually be very similar). The organs in the inner ear are beginning to develop, sending signals to his ever-expanding brain. Your little rocker first hears low-pitched sounds, so it's time to start talking to your baby, Dad!

Your baby is about the size of a pair of Bose headphones and weighs a little over a pound. So many things are growing and coming together, like the lungs. Blood vessels are expanding that will allow him to breathe. Your baby is making breathing movements, but this is just practice. Your wife's placenta is still acting as his oxygen mask. Those lungs won't be full of air until he's born. But when he does see the light of day . . . oh holy heck, will those lungs fill to release the raging and roaring otherwise known as crying.

CALL OF THE WILD

As a father, you'll need to differentiate the types of cries coming from your baby. And listen—babies cry a lot! But that's because it's the only way they know how to communicate. I read about research that shows babies are actually fantastic communicators. It found that 55 percent of all face-to-face communication comes from nonverbal signals such as facial expressions or body language, while 38 percent comes from how the words are said and only 7 percent comes from the actual words spoken.

So while babies can't articulate what they're thinking, they can wail and scream and sob and blubber. At this stage in their development, they really cry for only a few reasons. Here are the most common forms of baby bawls:

Annoyed and bored. This cry starts off as cooing as they try to interact and slowly turns to fussing. It's a slower, lower cry. Lots of whimpering and "What the heck, Dad? Just hold me and make that one weird face I like!"

Hangry. Yeah. That's right. They're not just hungry. They're ravenous. If your baby is fussy and you notice her putting her hands in her mouth, there's a good chance she's super hungry. This is usually a fast, rhythmic cry.

Tired. This is the lazy cry, the arm-stretching, mouth-yawning, eye-drooping fussing with a big "owww" sound. This is usually a slow, rhythmic cry. Best remedy for this is a good dad rock—no, not like Wilco. I mean actually rock your baby. Pick baby up and walk him around. Sometimes you even have to go outside for some natural white noise and fresh air.

Scared cry. You don't need to see *The Exorcist,* because when
babies are freaked out, they'll play you that film's soundtrack.
This cry is a shrill scream. It usually happens when your baby
gets startled. Maybe Dad gets a little too intense with
peekaboo. You'll know it when you hear it . . . This cry could
also signal pain. Maybe there is a binky in her car seat
jabbing her in the ribs. Also, wait until your baby gets the
stomach bug for the first time—much like *The Exorcist,* it
ain't pretty.

When it comes to understanding what babies are trying to tell us,
it's all about listening. They know exactly what they want, and they
ask for it. We just have to learn how to tune in.

TODDLER TANTRUMS

When babies become toddlers, their sobbing turns into tantrums.
This is where your kid loses his mind for seemingly no reason. He
just goes berserk. When you have a toddler, the only thing more
consistent than the sun coming up will be your kid having tantrums.

So why do kids throw tantrums? Is it because I'm a terrible parent?
That lady at the supermarket seems to think so! MIND YOUR
OWN BUSINESS, LINDA!

I'm going to let you in on a little secret. All toddlers throw tantrums. We've been giving them all they need their entire lives, as we
should, but at age sixteen months, they develop these things called
wants. The problem is, they think we're going to give them all they
want, too, which is why I have to keep reminding my kids of what
Mick Jagger said best.

"You can't always get what you want."

Now, the best way I've found to deal with tantrums is to stop
them before they start. All toddlers have triggers; for my kids, it's the
word *no.* So instead, I say no without actually saying no. "You can

have a popsicle, okay? Right after we have our lunch, we'll have popsicles." See what I did there? I just said no by saying yes.

Toddlers also tend to have tantrums whenever there's a transition. So if I just turn off the television and say "TV time is over," they're going to lose it. Instead, I give them a warning. "After this episode is done, we're going to go play Play-Doh." Now they know what's coming, and the rug's not pulled out from under them.

Another thing I do when one of our kids is about to go into a tantrum is to try to distract them. "Hey, look, look, look, look—what's this over here near the door? Is it the CAT? LOOK AT HIS FUNNY TAIL! OMG, HIS TAIL IS FUNNY!" Anything I can do to get them off that train wreck of a path they're about to get on, because once they're in tantrum mode, it's so hard to get them out of it. The tantrum is a train. Trains are hard to stop. The longer a tantrum goes on, the more momentum it has and the less chance there is of stopping the train wreck.

Tantrums are definitely one of the most draining, challenging things to deal with as a new parent. It's so easy for us to lose our patience and throw our own tantrum. Unfortunately, this will only increase the drama in the situation. It adds more train cars, but in a complicated, high-school-algebra sort of way. "If this train leaves the station at ninety miles per hour heading east and this train leaves the other station at seventy-five miles per hour heading west, where will they collide?" It sucks, but *we* have to be the adult. We have to hold it together to help them.

If you're not able to stop the tantrum before it starts, you're now in distract mode. Do whatever it takes to remove your kid from the situation and distract her. I've also found that the best time to address behavior and try to teach isn't always in the heat of the moment. If your kid is having a tantrum, she'll hear 0 percent of what you say. Instead, distract her, wait it out, and then try to talk to her. This is easier said than done. Tantrums are loud, and they're infuriating. They suck.

But . . . here's the silver lining—the cognitive limitations that make toddlers throw tantrums also make them curious and adventurous and just so much fun. They giggle when they see a turtle up close. They marvel at the wonder that is the car wash. They're fascinated by all the tiny things in life that we get to walk them through on a daily basis. Their tantrums have everything to do with their brains not being fully developed, but *we* get to be there and help them develop. We get to witness them tasting ice cream for the first time and help them catch their first frog. We get to teach them how to make a sandcastle and see the wonder in their eyes the first time it snows. Tantrums are hard, but once you learn a few Jedi mind tricks and when you look at all the joys and wonders of toddlerhood . . . it's so worth it.

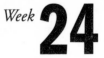

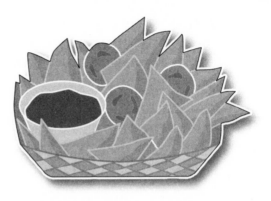

CONCESSION-STAND NACHOS

Yeah, that's right. I'm comparing your precious little nugget to some slimy pile of soggy chips slathered in hamburger and melted cheese. Come on—you know the kind I'm talking about. The kind you get in the hallway right outside the gymnasium where kids are attempting to play basketball.

Right now your baby is around twelve inches long from heel to head and weighs around 1.5 pounds. Organs and muscles are growing, and your budding jalapeño is putting on some baby fat, which helps steady the temperature gauge. And while he's already grown some hair, right now those little locks are white because of the lack of pigment in them.

If your baby were born right now, he could survive outside the uterus with the help of lots of care from doctors and nurses. According to the October 2017 issue of *Obstetrics & Gynecology* (a great publication—way better than *Popular Mechanics* or *Entertainment*

Weekly!), 42 to 59 percent of babies born at twenty-four weeks will be able to eventually go home with their families. This is remarkable when you consider that's just over halfway there.

Your wife might have developed a black line running down her belly. This is called the *linea nigra*. It's very normal and caused by (you guessed it) hormones.

This is like the time you woke up and found some black lines on your belly that say "It's My Life." You shouldn't worry either. This is just your favorite Bon Jovi song that you had tattooed on your tummy after the last guys' night out at Chili's. The linea nigra usually goes away several months after childbirth, but that bold, inked manifesto is yours forever.

DYNAMITE

I feel nostalgic every time I see concession-stand food. When I was a kid and played baseball every summer, my parents would give me a few bucks to spend on nachos or a hot dog after the game. The same went for all the wrestling meets we attended, and there were a lot of them since I wrestled all through grade school and middle school. I *dominated* youth wrestling. Partially because I was good, but also because in fifth grade I weighed only sixty pounds. Yeah, that's right—in fifth grade I weighed as much as one bag of cement. If you were going to pour a three-foot-deep footer for your porch, you would need three bags of me. To put that in perspective, the average fifth-grade male weighs eighty-five pounds.

Sure, I was small, but I was also very scrappy. My father loved to joke, "Dynamite comes in small packages." Because of my size, there usually weren't enough competitors to fill out a bracket for me at a wrestling tournament, so a lot of times I had to wrestle only one or two kids, and many of these were simply small and weak. I ended up dominating my size, and I grew accustomed to winning, which became a problem because I didn't learn how to lose.

I'll never forget winning the state wrestling tournament in the sixty-pound-bag-of-cement bracket. It isn't my victory that I remember the most; it's my dad's reaction. I'll never forget how he ran out onto the mat and grabbed me, then literally threw me up in the air because he was so excited and the adrenaline was pumping through him. He was just as thrilled as I was, if not more, because he was so proud of his son.

When I got older and my competition grew tougher, wrestling became hard for me. Before every match, I became increasingly anxious. I would get all worked up with so much anxiety that the sport wasn't fun any longer. Eventually I quit. I felt a tremendous amount of shame because I knew my dad didn't want me to quit and I felt I was disappointing him, though he never said that. He let me quit because that's what I wanted to do, and that's when I became interested in acting. I ended up entering every high school play I could, and when I went to college, I performed in ten productions. My parents came to every one. Musicals, dramas, comedies—it didn't matter; they were always there.

After one of those plays in college, my dad told me that every night I performed, he felt like he was watching me win the state wrestling tournament. He was so proud of me, and he could see how being in those productions made me feel. How they gave me an adrenaline rush and confidence and how being in them was so fulfilling.

I think that, at the end of the day, the thing we as kids want more than anything else is just our fathers' approval. When I decided I didn't want to wrestle anymore, I was so scared to tell my dad because I was nervous he would be disappointed. But when he shared with me how he felt watching me in those theater productions, I felt elated, knowing I had his approval. I also realized that he simply wanted to see me doing something that made me feel fulfilled and proud, something that gave me joy. I didn't have to do something grandiose to earn his approval. He just wanted me to be happy.

As a father myself, I now have a chance to be the one expressing pride and affirmation. Whether it's sitting in the stands at a wrestling match or in a seat for a performance, I get to celebrate my children and see what fills them with pride and joy. I can applaud their achievements and accept their decisions, wherever they might lead.

The word *champion* is a noun that refers to someone who wins first prize in a competition. But *champion* is also a verb that means to support and defend and fight for a person or belief or principle. It's natural for a father to want his kids to be champions. But as fathers, we always need to champion our children in whatever path they take.

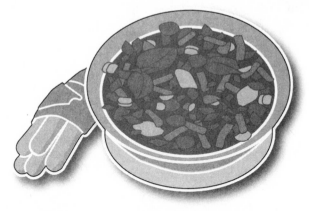

BOWL OF OLIVE GARDEN SOUP AND BREADSTICKS

It's near the end of the second trimester, so it's time to celebrate by taking your wife to Olive Garden! She has now become too familiar with feeling constipated and bloated, so why not binge at America's favorite Italian restaurant? That way you'll have as much gas as she does! Overeating will also probably give you indigestion, so you can just tell your wife you're suffering right alongside her.

At week 25, the baby's nostrils are opening up, so imagine your little nugget smelling the sweet aroma of alfredo sauce. Baby's hands are now fully formed, but they're much smaller than yours, so they'll have to wait awhile before they can double fist breadsticks. By now the baby is about the size of a bowl of soup and those breadsticks—roughly 13.5 inches from the top of her head to the bottom of her feet, which is exactly the size your belly is going to feel after those five bowls of soup.

So here's some looking-down-the-road perspective, dad to dad.

Some things in your life as a parent are going to be as endless as the soup and breadsticks at Olive Garden. The diapers will be endless. The tears will be endless. The giggles and the fights and the mealtime negotiations will be endless, so it will be impossible to not slip into a routine. It's going to be way too easy for you and your spouse to get stuck in that nightly routine where you put the kids down and then stare at your phones for a couple of hours before going to bed. You're gonna be too exhausted to do anything else.

We all fall into the rut of routines. Even when we go to Olive Garden, we open that menu, thinking, *I'm going to get something different,* but we never do. You contemplate ordering the Five Cheese Ziti al Forno, but then you end up going with the soup and breadsticks just like the last hundred times. The Zuppa Toscana is familiar and comfortable, so you just go with it.

I challenge you to *occasionally* break the routine.

Now, as a parent, routine is your friend. It can be extremely helpful because the more routine you have, the more your kids will know what to expect and the better behaved they'll be because they know their boundaries. But I challenge you to occasionally break that routine. When you set a good schedule, switching it up can be a great way to make an impact on your kids.

My mom was the queen of breaking up routines. When I was a kid, on the first nice spring day when the weather shifted and it became gorgeous outside, I'd find myself waking up with warm sunlight streaming into my bedroom. I'd be wondering what had happened, knowing it wasn't 7:30 A.M., and then I'd check the clock and discover it was 10:00. I'd find my mom outside and ask her what was going on.

"It's too nice to go to school," she'd say. "You're staying home."

I'd smile and think, *All right, I just got a full day off.*

"I already called the school and let them know you're not coming in. Now spend the day outside," my mom would tell me.

Every now and then as a parent, you're going to need to change things up. Your kids will never expect it. It might take them a minute to even process what's happening. Be brave and bold. But remember . . . you have to have routines in place in order to be able to sometimes break away from them.

Since you don't have to call the school's front office just yet, why don't you take a big leap of faith the next time you're at Olive Garden? Maybe it's finally time for you to take the Tour of Italy. I know you're going to Olive Garden soon, because you can't talk about the soup and breadsticks this long and not want to go get them.

*Olive Garden: Not a sponsor. (Yet!)

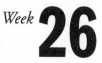

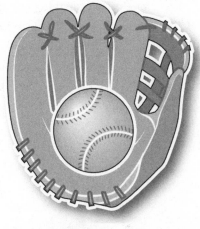

BASEBALL GLOVE

Little dude is now the size of a baseball glove. Remember when you got a brand-new baseball glove and needed to oil it and massage the leather to break it in? Your wife's back now needs the same attention. She's likely experiencing some back pain due to the two-pound human currently growing inside her, which is at least 50 percent your fault. So give your lady a good ole back rub. The key to a good back rub is being fully present and always mixing it up. Don't let her muscles know what's coming next. Just when she thinks you're about to go thumbs to the lower back—*bam*—hit her with a forehead bounce to the shoulder blades. Trust me, she'll love it.

Your baby is starting to open his eyes now, and his hand coordination is also improving. These are necessary since one day you'll be playing catch with your kid and teaching him how to throw a curveball. Even if he never becomes a pitcher, it's always good for bragging rights.

As a dad, playing with your kids is part of your job. Men can have youthful spirits that make us, well . . . more fun to kids. Whether you're throwing a baseball or blowing bubbles or dressing up Barbie dolls, this is Dad's domain. But like anything else, it's a bit of an acquired skill, and if you've never been around babies or toddlers before, you might not know how to best interact. You can't exactly teach them to throw a curve when they're two. But you definitely can play with them! Here are some tips I've compiled on how to play with little kids, toddlers, and even babies:

1. **Be an idiot.** You can't be self-conscious. Let loose and let the goof out. "Grow up. Be a man!" they say. I say, "Who cares?" Your kids certainly couldn't care less. The same buffoonery that won your wife over will win your kids over tenfold.

2. **Anticipation.** The buildup is 90 percent of the game. If you tell them you'll tickle them, you'll get them laughing long before you reach them. It's like a good suspense movie. Tell them to go hide, and take forever to find them even though you see their little feet plain as day sticking out from under the rug.

3. **Repetition.** It might get old, but they love repetition. It's actually an important part of development. You might find yourself reading the same book fifteen times in a row. Stick with it! Through repetition, possibilities become abilities.

4. **Let them lead.** It's okay to guide them and teach them, but at the end of the day, you're there to have fun. So if you really want to play catch but they want to throw the ball out of the tree house and make you chase it, why fight it? Go fetch the ball.

5. **Just look at them.** Pay attention. Playtime is all about connection. Even a baby is affected by eye contact and a goofy smile. It doesn't matter if you can do the perfect Donald

Duck voice or if you're the most completely straitlaced guy in the world. Your kids don't care. These days won't last forever. Your kids are going to be begging you to play with them, but you're going to be staring at your phone, and then one day you're going to look up and they won't be there . . . and you'll be begging them to hang out with you. I get emotional about it because I'm just as guilty as everybody else. Honestly, it's partially just because we're so flippin' tired. We're so worn out from doing everything we can to keep them alive that we don't feel like we have the energy to do *this* part of it. Which is just as important, if not more important, to them. So put down your phone, go find your kids, and act like a goofball.

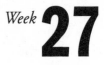

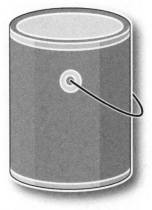

GALLON OF PAINT

A one-gallon can of paint? Really? I know what you're thinking: *Isn't that a stretch, Dr. Calmus?* But consider the size, not necessarily the weight. Imagine that you and your wife have already used most of the paint in the can while painting the nursery pink or blue. Or maybe you're going to be rebellious and just douse it with an avant-garde neon green. Little one is going to love whatever color you pick.

This is a room where cherished memories will be made. A place of blissful love and peaceful parenting. A quiet place to read baby books and rock her to sleep. A sanctuary full of sunshine and rainbows. An alcove that will keep out the storms.

Now that we're done painting the room, let me paint you an honest picture. You've seen those smiley snapshots your friends post with their kids on social media? The ones where they're smiling in a pumpkin patch and they're all in matching attire? You know, the ones that depict their lives as all sunshine and rainbows? Let me help redirect your expectations . . . Those pics are mostly full of it. But someday soon you'll be doing the same thing. Doesn't make you a bad person. It's what everybody does. Sure, it can create unrealistic expectations, but it also allows everyone to share in your joyful moments. We post the sweet and happy memories while we tend to pass over the crummy and frustrating moments.

Those moments are inevitable, though.

Waking up at one in the morning, then at two, then at three.

Listening to your kid wail for no reason.

Finding Sharpie doodles on your brand-new dresser.

Endlessly telling your kid to put his shoes on.

There are days that turn bad before you even have breakfast. You won't have had a chance to burn toast yet, and your patience will be gone. It will be the only thing that gets you out the door on time—your patience.

Some days are so frustrating that you'll want to put your kid to bed at four o'clock in the afternoon. You'll want to just hop in the car and drive anywhere by yourself without the sound of a screaming toddler or "Baby Shark" (it's honestly tough to tell which is worse).

The *screaming*. So much screaming. ALWAYS SCREAMING . . . The screaming will be endless and will follow you everywhere.

Being a dad is extremely rewarding sometimes, but other times doing the right thing means that your kid is probably going to hate you for a while. You'll have a fight because you won't let him eat cat food. And you and your wife will also fight. Like every couple before you, you'll *fight* (and probably fight more after having kids than you did before). And sometimes you'll feel so disconnected that you try to blame your problems on each other.

You'll feel like you can't do anything right. Not a single dang thing. You'll feel like a failure.

Yes, fatherhood is hard, but if you allow yourself to be exhausted all the time, you're going to *miss it*.

At some point your kid will be obsessed with playing hide-and-seek with you. So every night, he'll beg to play it. You'll have just gotten home, and you will be tired and will just want to check out.

Do it anyway. Parenting is a selfless task, and if you don't operate with that mentality, everyone loses.

Your child will be chasing you through the house, and you'll both be screaming like idiots. And it's that same annoying scream, but now you appreciate it because he's not trying to be annoying. He's expressing how much he loves spending time with you. He's expressing how much he loves you.

Then you'll be hiding again in the most obvious place, and somehow your little kid can't find you, but your wife sees you, and you lock eyes. You know exactly what she's thinking, because you're thinking the same thing. And in that moment, you'll feel more connected than ever without even saying a single word.

Your life will be sunshine and rainbows. But that doesn't mean that a storm didn't just pass through or that another storm won't come tomorrow.

Just like we choose what we post on social media, we can choose what we focus on in our lives.

Things She'll Say During the **Third** Trimester

"Holy cow, I'm winded . . . all because I just put my pants on."

"AAAGGGHHH. IF THIS BABY DOESN'T COME OUT OF ME THIS WEEK, I'M GOING TO BURN THIS WHOLE PLACE DOWN! I WANT MY BODY BACK."

"Oh, the baby's kicking! The baby's kicking! Watch. Watch. You see that?"

"Get your foot off my ribs, baby."

"Stop kicking my bladder!"

"What? It's my belly balm. If I don't use this twice a day, I'm going to look like a deflated beach ball. You want that? Hmmm? Hmmm?"

"Oh, these Braxton-Hicks are fuh-real."

"You better be cute, because you're seriously ruining your mommy's body. You hear me? I used to be a golden goddess."

"Babe, do you still find me attractive? Why are you not answering? You don't want to answer. I KNOW WHAT YOU'RE THINKING! YOU DID THIS!"

"Are you head down? You better be head down. If you make your mommy get a C-section, I'm going to name you something stupid like Sheesh."

"Oh my gosh, babe, our baby weighs twenty-two pounds. I mean, that has got to be the baby's weight. That is not my weight."

"Hold on. I'm Instagramming my stretch marks. Shut up. People want to see this on my feed—it's empowering."

"Babe, my water just broke. Wait . . . Never mind. It's just pee. I just peed myself again."

"All right, I am motivated today. Mama is going to do some nesting . . . zzzzzzz."

"I feel like a cheap motel, except I provide breakfast and everyone keeps peeing in the pool."

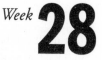
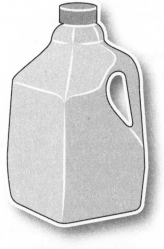

MILK JUG

Your baby dude is now the size of a jug of milk. Speaking of jugs, *my wife's boobs are so freaking enormous right now!* I mean, seriously! They say when the baby comes, I'll have to share her breasts with the baby. Honestly, I'm totally cool with that because there is enough to go around! They. Are. Massive. And none of her clothes are built to handle the extra mammary load, so those puppies are just busting out.

Ready for some pregnancy facts? Your baby is waking and sleeping according to a somewhat-regular cycle now, and his breathing and yawning are becoming more regular too. As for Mom, she's probably going to the doctor every couple of weeks now for checkups and ultrasounds. Remember! Mom will likely want you at as many of these appointments as possible, so try to block and tackle your schedule ahead of time.

Also, my wife's boobs are overflowing and everywhere, and I can't stop thinking about those bazookas. Sorry, I'm super distracted right now. But speaking about breasts and milk reminds me of some helpful info I've acquired watching my wife nurse. I'd like to call this segment "Breastfeeding Dude-splained."

BREASTFEEDING DUDE-SPLAINED

Breastfeeding is crazy because moms become instantly responsible for the life of a human being. I mean, you're responsible, too, but Mom's got a real competitive advantage here. Sometimes her milk supply doesn't come in for like two to three days after your baby is born. So for the first three days, you're just like, "What do I feed 'em?" Usually Mom's body is still making colostrum at this point, which is basically nutrient-rich pre-milk. It's like a protein shake chock full of antibodies for your new baby.

Now, when the milk does finally come in, it's going to make her breasts swell several times larger—like the Grinch's heart. Pause to applaud, but be forewarned. She'll be in a lot of discomfort. She might even feel stabbing pain . . . as if Kylo Ren were having an emo fit, just light-sabering everything in sight, but the control panel of the Star Destroyer is actually just the inside of her breasts. So listen— there are things called heat/ice packs. Throw one in the freezer so she can ice her bosom, or throw it in the microwave so she can heat her bosom. "Hot or cold, your wish is my command, dear!"

One of the most important early moments in breastfeeding is establishing a good latch. It's like all the people in those Subway commercials; they don't take just a normal sandwich bite. It's always like a massive bite devouring half the sub. That's how your baby needs to latch. If he's having trouble latching, you can help your wife get an appointment with a lactation consultant. Yes, there are literally experts whose entire job is to help babies and moms with their latch. I know what you're thinking: *This is kinda weird.* Yeah, it is, but you've got to put on your big boy pants and talk with compassion and kindness about all sorts of stuff that makes the junior higher living inside you want to snicker.

Okay, guys, so you know how when you work a really long, hard day after not having worked with your hands in a while, you get all these blisters and calluses? This might happen to your wife's nipples. So to help with her sore, cracked nipples, she should use nipple butter. What doesn't butter make better? I mean—corn on the cob, toast, mashed potatoes, nipples.

Another great thing to help out with raw nipples is Silverette cups. They're like tiny metal hats that your wife can put on her nipples. It's like that thimble from Monopoly—the piece no one wants . . . until now. They're made out of actual silver, which has healing properties that will relieve your wife's nipples. They'll also act as a shield and prevent rubbing against her bra. Again, file this in the "things I never thought I'd be reading about" category of your brain. But I'm glad you are. You probably don't need to suggest any of these cures to your wife, but it's good to be knowledgeable so that you can lend a hand and help find the right stuff.

Now, before we get too deep into this breastfeeding conversation, let me just say this . . . There are plenty of mommy blogs out there arguing about breastfeeding versus formula, and this book is not that. This is just one dude talking to another dude to help him better understand his wife during this life-changing experience. With that said, here are the pros and cons of breastfeeding.

PROS

Breastfeeding can give your baby stronger bones, a lower SIDS risk, and fewer problems with weight. It will help your wife regain some of her own hormonal balance. It's cheap. Not only does breastfeeding save you money on formula, but it's also liquid gold. You can sell breast milk for one to five dollars an ounce online. Your wife's boobs are making it rain money. Breast milk is also fine-tuned to your baby's needs. Your baby's saliva will work its way into the nipple and tell your wife's body what the baby needs in the milk to make her feel better if she's sick. Yeah, your wife's nipples are like a baby nutritionist and pharmacist rolled into one.

CONS

Breastfeeding is also a *ton* of work and isn't always feasible for every mom. Moms burn two hundred to five hundred extra calories every day just by producing milk. This can leave them feeling extremely fatigued. Some women also have challenges producing milk, and other times a baby just doesn't want to latch. A mother and her baby begin to form a feeding schedule together, and if that schedule gets interrupted, it can throw off her milk supply. Some moms have responsibilities that require them to be away from their baby during feeding times, which means they'll have to pump. They literally have to hook themselves to a machine, or they'll become engorged and sore and will potentially stop producing milk. There are many reasons that some moms choose to use formula. This is one of those areas where it's best for us to let them make the decision, and we as dads should just support them and our kiddos however we can!

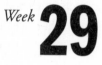
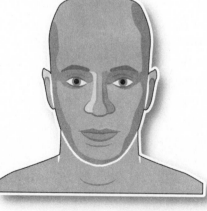

HUMAN HEAD

Some say your baby right now is as big as a butternut squash, and others claim your son or daughter is the size of a head of cauliflower. But forget pumpkins and cruciferous vegetables. We're going with a human head! And that's not weird at all!

And while we're talking about heads, your baby's head is continuing to grow rapidly to house his ever-developing brain. From this week until birth, your baby's cerebrum will triple in weight! And since the head is the heaviest part of your baby, gravity and the shape of Mommy's uterus *usually* get him into the head-down position.

At around fifteen to sixteen inches and two and a half to three pounds, your little Einstein is filling up Mom's womb. Those kicks your wife used to feel are now going to be nudges and jabs coming from knees and elbows. *Sweep the leg!*

Speaking of the brain, your wife's noodle might be feeling a little wonky these days (a fact to be aware of but perhaps not to offer as a fun talking point over dinner with friends). Being stressed, not sleeping, and carrying a baby can lead to forgetfulness. But it's not just that. It's raging hormones that are simmering her brain. Can you imagine how scatterbrained we would be if dads were the ones doing the heavy lifting of pregnancy? Jeesh. We already have trouble multitasking. Additionally, when it's time to deliver the baby, the same oxytocin that makes your wife's uterus contract and her breasts produce milk also starts short-circuiting her brain (possibly to provide some mental distance from the pain of childbirth).

So, guys . . . "momnesia" is a real thing. Be gentle if she forgets things. And help fill in the gaps where you can!

THE DAD SOFA

Remember the famous line from the 1931 film *Frankenstein* when the titular character shouts, "It's alive. It's moving. It's alive; it's alive; it's alive; it's alive. It's alive!" This is how you're going to feel when you first see that head popping out of your wife during delivery. Sure, the top of my son's head did resemble a wet muskrat squeezing out of the small hole in his pond hut . . . Okay, maybe don't picture that.

With our first delivery, I was binge-watching *Making a Murderer* around midnight when Heidi called out from the bathroom.

"I think my water broke, but I'm not sure because I peed in it."

As I drove her to the hospital, I timed her contractions and calculated that they were three minutes apart. At least, I thought they were, but I'd never done this before, so I had no idea if I was doing it right. After arriving at the hospital, I became upset at the complete lack of urgency while my wife was in pain. While Heidi grimaced and groaned, some nurse gave me a form to fill out and suggested I have a seat. It was almost like they'd gone through this sort of thing before.

So my wife was struggling with all this pain, and I just sat there feeling helpless. If I could have grown a uterus and had the baby for her, I absolutely would have. But I couldn't. When she became dilated far enough, we were able to move into labor and delivery. We were there for hours, giving me the chance to watch a couple more episodes of *Making a Murderer* while my very pregnant wife took a much-needed drug-induced nap. I ended up spending lots of time lounging on what they call "the dad sofa." It's what guys use for a bed, but it's not an actual foldout sofa—they just give you another couch cushion to sleep on. So in essence, they should call it "the crappy couch."

When it came time for Heidi to start pushing, I felt like I was part coach ("You got this, Heidi—you can do this!") and part yoga instructor ("Okay, just put your leg on my right shoulder there and take several deep breaths").

The real question facing most dads at this point is whether they want to stay above the curtain (top half of Mom-to-be) or below the curtain (bottom half of Mom-to-be). This is a big decision, especially if you're a little squeamish. It's probably good to think about this moment ahead of time and talk strategy as a couple. It's absolutely magical to see your little one emerge into the world, but it's also very medically and biologically *intense.* So you have to know yourself a bit and make a good decision from there. You can always run the option, but it's good to have a plan A.

THE MOMENT OF TRUTH

You're probably wondering all sorts of things about the delivery, about what's going to happen and what you're going to see. Is it a little gross? Definitely. Did it freak me out? No, because, in that moment, I wasn't thinking about sex. And I was confident that the doctors were taking good care of Heidi. Instead, I was thinking, *Holy schnikes, there's a baby in there, and he's coming out, and that's my kid, and like, holy smokes, I have a kid! Oh my gosh. That's his head? Oh my gosh, he has a head! He's amazing!* I've heard a lot of dads say they were so high on adrenaline that the biological stuff didn't freak them out. They were completely dialed in, like on game day, ready to love their lady and meet their kiddo.

The only thing certain in birth is that nothing is certain. My wife pushed to physical exhaustion for an hour and a half with our first son before the doctor had to attach a suction cup tool to the top of little Theo's head and tug-of-war him out. Then nineteen months later when we had our daughter, the doctor walked in and asked if Heidi could try pushing. Heidi pushed twice, and the doctor said, "Okay, that's good. Now just cough."

Cough.

"Waaaahhhh."

Just like that, baby Juno was born.

Our third baby, Otto, was a mix of the first two. He was late, so we finally went into the hospital to get induced, and then before we could do that, labor kicked in all at once. By the time the anesthesiologist arrived to give Heidi an epidural, it was too late. It was already time to push. She held a helium-fed mask to her face and screamed into it as she pushed. She was loopy from the helium and couldn't hear the doctor over her own screaming, so I became relay man shouting at her from two feet away. The doctor would yell, "Take a deep breath!" Then I would yell, "Take a deep breath!" The doctor would shout, "Put your chin down and push!" Then I would shout, "Put your chin down and push!" I continued repeating everything the doctor yelled for the next ten minutes before beautiful baby Otto was born.

Perhaps labor and delivery will feel like endless hours of waiting, or perhaps it will feel like a whirlwind and you won't remember a thing. Maybe you're going to want to know every grisly medical detail, or maybe you simply won't want to look behind the curtain (totally fine!). Maybe things will become difficult enough that the doctor will need to perform an episiotomy or an emergency C-section (hang tight—y'all are gonna make it!).

You'll be there seeing your child for the first time. Feeling that little hand grab your pinkie and finding something in your brain opening for the very first time. Getting to hold her and say her name as she opens her eyes to see a very blurry version of you.

Even though you and your lady are incredibly tired, try hard to be present for this very special moment. This is the moment when you know that nothing in your life is ever going to be the same. It's the moment you become a dad.

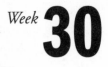
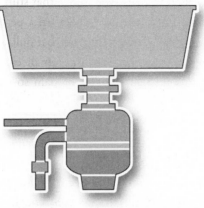

GARBAGE DISPOSAL

Hey, dude. Do me a favor. Go to your kitchen. Yeah, take this book along. That's one fun thing about being in a book. You can take me anywhere.

Okay, so open the cupboard underneath the sink. Chances are you have a garbage disposal under one of the drains. You know—the three-quarters-horsepower thing that resembles a canister. This is the size of your baby right now in Mommy's incubator. Very soon you'll be throwing his uneaten mashed pea puree or barely nibbled hot dog sticks into that very same disposal.

The great thing about a garbage disposal is that it gets rid of all the extra stuff in your kitchen. The crust of a PB&J sandwich left over on a Dora the Explorer plate. The skin of a potato you just peeled. The leftover spaghetti sauce that's developed fuzzy mold in the fridge. When in doubt, just plop it in the sink, turn on the water, and flip the disposal's switch on.

As you look ahead to becoming a dad, now is a good time to start discarding the garbage around you. In a material sense, this means cleaning out the room that will be used for the nursery and scrapping stuff you haven't used in years (you know, that stuff still in boxes in the guest bedroom from your *last* move). In a personal sense, this means cleaning out the unnecessary stuff that pulls on your time or pushes on your priorities—like all that email cluttering up your inbox, it's time to send that straight to spam so you can be more nimble when baby comes!

What's the small stuff in your life that you're currently sweating? All those minor annoyances that collectively become a major burden. Here's the thing—when your little one arrives, there's only going to be more small stuff. Literally (Legos and Cheerios and SpaghettiOs) and figuratively (our daughter has a slight cough . . . OH NO! IS SHE COMING DOWN WITH EBOLA?). But the thing is, you have some time before parenthood begins. So why not tidy up your life now?

Start by asking yourself the following question: *What are the drains on my time and energy that I need to dispose of right now?*

Imagine your life as a kitchen. It starts sparse with shiny appliances, sparkling counters, and the smell of fresh paint. Over time you fill the cabinets and drawers with bowls and blenders and utensils and pots and pans. Some remain unused while others start to fall apart. Your burners start to rust. Your fridge starts to stink. And God forbid anybody dares to look underneath that stove! Meanwhile, all day long, you're throwing things away, but sometimes the garbage disposal gets clogged up. Sometimes the dishes don't get cleaned. Sometimes there are so many crumbs in your kitchen that the casts of both *A Bug's Life* and *Antz* come to visit.

We can get so overloaded on living that our pantries and cupboards become packed with useless trinkets and junk. Our fridge is full of forgotten leftovers—do *not* eat that tuna fish salad. This is the stuff we need to discard. Social media binges. Stressing about politics and world events. Keeping up with the Joneses. Concern about our 401(k).

What needs to be shoved down that disposal, ground up, and sent down the drain?

FORGETTING TO HAVE FUN

"Don't sweat the small stuff" isn't just a nice catchphrase; it's also the title of one of the fastest-selling books of all time. Released in 1997, *Don't Sweat the Small Stuff* became *USA Today*'s bestselling book for two straight years and spent more than a hundred weeks on *The New York Times* bestseller list.

Richard Carlson stressed how to live a stress-free life. His gift to others was the freedom he found in not letting trivial things take over. Here's a great quote from *Don't Sweat the Small Stuff* that can apply to anyone but applies especially well to parents:

> I've never met anyone (myself included) who hasn't turned little things into great big emergencies. We take our own goals so seriously that we forget to have fun along the way, and we forget to cut ourselves some slack. We take simple preferences and turn them into conditions for our own happiness. Or, we beat ourselves up if we can't meet our self-created deadlines.

So what are those little things that can turn into lifelong headaches and heartburn? Your kid scratched your new car. The house is a mess. Your son got called into the principal's office. Can you forgive and forget? Do you have to clean up? Are you going to hold a grudge?

At the end of the day, what are the things that truly matter? What can be cut out of your life and disposed of?

Whenever I notice that my day is extra stressful, I try to step away from my circumstances, fly a metaphorical hot-air balloon two thousand feet up, look down on myself, and think, *Will this thing I'm worried about matter in five years? How about five months? Five days? Or can I shrug this off and be happy with everything in my life that is going right?*

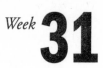

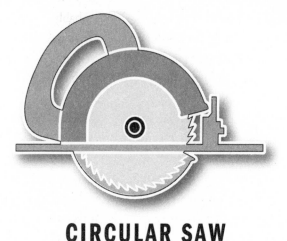

CIRCULAR SAW

Only nine more weeks to go! Right now your baby is three pounds and around sixteen inches long and is about the size of a circular saw. The baby's brain is spinning like the blade on a circular saw as it continues to build billions of new connections. Your baby can use all five of her senses, so if you're busy building something for her in your garage, she might hear the noise from inside her little cave.

By now you might be tired of the endless advice you and especially your wife have been hearing. But let me offer some of the best I've heard. My dad has only one piece of advice for new parents: "You have to let your kid fall out of trees." I remember him always saying this, and I also remember my siblings and me falling out of a lot of trees. It's so short and simple, but it's difficult to live out. Now, he's not encouraging parents to let their kids do reckless things; he's encouraging parents to give their kids room to learn independence and have their own adventures. My dad built many things, including a batting cage and a tree house, so that we could have adventures.

I'll never forget that old tree house. I don't think there was a new piece of lumber on it anywhere. It wasn't big—it must have been only five feet long by five feet wide—and it probably stood about five feet off the ground. It had doors on each side as well as a trap door that we fell out of sometimes. There was even a rope swing! We usually ended up swinging out and then right back into the side of the tree house wall. *Bang!*

My dad decided to put in a zip line that would carry us from another tree over to the tree house. I'm glad there aren't building inspectors for zip lines, because they definitely wouldn't have liked this setup. We had to climb ten feet straight up a ladder that wasn't angled even a bit. We then had to keep our balance while turning around at the top of the ladder in order to face the zip line. After grabbing a little handle, we jumped and slid down the zip line, which was hooked directly to the side of the tree house. We'd come flying in and try to put our feet up before slamming into the wall of old barn wood. After bouncing back about four feet, we'd simply let go and drop four feet to the ground.

Looking back, I don't think my dad even tried to make that tree house safe. When he first hooked up the zip line, he wrapped the end of the line to a big tree. My brother, being the older, smarter one, took one look at the zip line and told me I should try it out first. So I, being the younger brother that I was, tried it and promptly slammed into the tree before falling on my back. My brother then suggested that we might need to change the setup.

Though my father wasn't the handiest guy around, he did a lot of work with his hands and wasn't afraid to try things like building our tree house. And I'm so grateful, because we spent every day in that thing. There wasn't a kid in the entire school that had a tree house like ours. When my brother and I aged out of the tree house, our dad revamped it for our sister, who is nine years younger than me. He made it into a little girl's playhouse, complete with vinyl siding on the whole thing. Eventually the tree died and the entire structure fell over in a huge pile of memories.

My dad built a lot of that tree house using his circular saw. The thing about the circular saw is that it's not the most specialized tool for every job but it's a tool you can use for *almost* every job. For instance, if you want to do a miter cut, you're better off using a miter saw to get that nice, clean angled cut, but you *can* use a circular saw. It'll get the job done for you—just not as easily and maybe not as precisely. The same goes if you want to cut a long piece of plywood. You're better off using a table saw because you can run it along the fence to get a good, straight cut, but that means you'd have to go to the trouble of pulling the table saw out of the garage. The easier solution is simply using a circular saw. It won't be as straight of a cut, but it'll get the job done.

It's the jack-of-all-trades of saws. I've always thought that my dad is like a circular saw because he's not an expert on any one thing but he can get the job done.

We should all strive to be circular saws in parenting our kids. Don't let your lack of expertise dissuade you from getting the job done.

You don't have to know how to perfectly coach a baseball team; you just have to coach. You don't have to know how to make a *Super Dad*-quality tree house; you just have to spend the time to make a solid tree house. You don't have to know how to fly-fish like Brad Pitt from *A River Runs Through It;* you just have to take your kids fishing and show them how to put a worm on the hook. You don't have to be an expert on anything; you just have to do the best job you can. Your kids aren't going to remember if you were an expert; they're just going to remember that you showed up when it counted.

Be the circular saw. Be the dad that is willing to take on any challenge to give your kids an experience even if you don't know exactly how. Strap on the tool belt and create the adventure. Be willing to step outside your comfort zone. At the end of the day, you're not just building a safe-ish tree house or swing set—you're building memories.

HOW TO ASSEMBLE *ANY* KIDS' TOY

1. Grab a beer. Now you're ready.
2. Dump hardware in pile.
3. Find instructions and burn them. You don't need those. You're a man.
4. Assemble it. Boom—done.
5. Throw excess hardware in junk drawer. (Why do they always send extra?)
6. Show wife completed project.
7. Try to convince wife that it's assembled correctly and that it's *perfectly safe.*
8. Try to salvage burnt instructions.
9. Try to find instructions online.
10. Try to connect to Wi-Fi.
11. Reset your router.
12. Call internet provider.
13. Find instructions online.
14. Disassemble it.
15. Reassemble it.
16. Break something.
17. Find a replacement part.
18. Make a beer run.
19. Assemble it one last time.
20. Conduct product testing.
21. Watch child instantly lose interest in the toy and play in the box it came in.

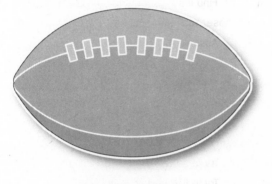

FOOTBALL

Your baby's face is almost completely developed, with eyelashes and eyebrows and even a little hair! Turn the music up to eleven, because his inner ears are formed and his lungs are getting ready to sing along. "Welcome to the Juuuungle!" He has plenty of room to dance since Mommy's uterus is about the size of a soccer ball, which fits nicely with our object this week since soccer outside the United States is called football. Your little baby is now around the length of an American football, or, as I call it, the ole pigskin.

Kids come in all shapes and sizes and personalities just like you find on the roster of a professional football team. In the NFL, every position is important, whether the player is rushing with the ball on offense or rushing the quarterback on defense, and in a similar way, every child is amazing and valuable with his own unique gifts and talents.

Some children are natural-born leaders, talented and decisive like a quarterback. They take charge and lead the team down the field or maybe just lead their friends into the sandbox to play.

Maybe you'll have an oddball child, someone who always surprises you. He's a lot like a free safety—he might be anywhere on the field at any time, striking when you don't expect it.

Perhaps you have a relentless Energizer Bunny of a child that never stops moving, that just keeps going and going. This means you have a defensive tackle, a player who keeps pushing and pushing until he gets a sack.

Maybe baby will be a perfectionist with laser-like precision, someone who follows the rules and knows the exact path to take. If so, you might have a wide receiver on your hands. Or actually in your hands.

What if your child is a bit of a lone ranger, someone who wants to do his own thing? An artist, a free spirit, moody, flighty, sometimes exasperating, and usually good under pressure. Yeah—you know who I'm talking about . . . The poor, long-suffering, "I get no respect" kicker.

As a father, you're the head coach. Whether you have one kid or ten, it doesn't matter. The rules remain the same. You can't execute *for* your players, but you can help get their heads in the game. In a similar fashion, once you become a student of your kid's talents and abilities, you can try to maximize them. If your kiddo is made to be a punter, don't keep forcing him to be a tight end because that was your position. And when you have multiple kids, help them play their own positions in light of their unique gifts and talents. As they get older, you'll get to direct the plays and guide them on the field of life.

So who exactly is your wife in this analogy?

Naturally she's the owner of the team. And ultimately she's the one doing all the recruiting. She calls the shots . . . which means, at any given time, she can fire you.

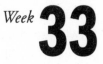

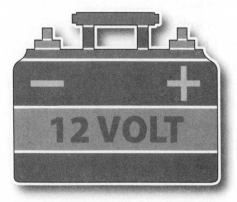

CAR BATTERY

For the past seven months, your wife has been experiencing different levels of fatigue as your baby has been growing. Why? One big reason is that her body has been providing oxygen and nutrients to your little dude. Think of your baby as an astronaut floating in space and your wife as the architect and construction crew for baby's space station. Not only does her placenta have a fully functional cafeteria, but it also ejects waste from little Buzz Lightyear's blood!

Another reason for the fatigue is that all systems and controls in the mother ship are out of whack. Heart rate is up and blood sugar is down. Hormones have reached critical level. Metabolism is blistering every ounce of energy produced.

These two reasons plus a thousand others are why the dame of the house might feel drained. Meanwhile, your little Energizer—about the size of a car battery—is almost fully developed, with lungs almost complete.

I'm sure there are times you feel for your wife, wishing you could support her like the dream pillow she sleeps on. You may not be able to precisely understand how drained she feels, but fear not, dear friend. Very soon you, too, will stand on the shores of sleepiness and stupor after your baby is born. FedEx is going to be bringing you a big package of exhaustion in about seven weeks (or maybe even sooner). You're going to wish that you ran on batteries, that you could simply be plugged in at the end of the day and recharged. But no amount of caffeine coursing through your veins will fill your tank all the way.

A lot of parenting is about pushing through all the fatigue. There will be days when your brain isn't going to work like it used to. There might be times when you can't seem to get your stuff together. You might miss a morning meeting, forget to take the stroller to the grocery store, or call one of your kids the wrong name.

You're going to have these days when you feel like you're running at 25 percent. Like you're just going through the motions. It will feel like nothing is going right, and you'll be so drained that when you pull into the driveway after work, you won't get out of your car. You might sit there alone just to enjoy a few more minutes of silence while you collect yourself and muster up the energy to walk inside. Then you'll look down and realize all the warning lights are on in your car, and you'll sigh and mentally add it to the growing list of things you need to get done.

Here's the thing, though. You'll also need to realize what a freaking legend you are. That mental list of stuff you need to get done will be so long it would have crippled you five years ago, but now it's just your norm. And you handle it! Your capacity to multitask will make you feel invincible, and you'll do it all on limited sleep. Parents don't get sick days. There will be days you feel like death, and you'll still find strength enough to take on the world. Also, dad strength is real! No CrossFit workout will build the same strength as carrying a sleeping toddler out of an amusement park to a parking lot four states away. Another thing that will make you feel like a superhero? Dad reflexes. You've seen the viral videos of dads grabbing their kids a split second before they catch a basketball to the face. You'll soon possess dad reflexes. I don't know how it works—maybe it's the way we're wired, maybe it's spiritual intuition, or maybe we develop a sixth sense—but you'll develop dad reflexes, and you'll save your children from severe pain on a multitude of occasions. And you'll feel like a legend, and it will keep you going. It will keep you charged.

TEACHABLE MOMENTS

Teach your kids how to jump-start a car. It's an easy task that *everyone* should know how to do. Not just your sons—your daughters too. If you yourself don't know how, google it. There are a billion instructional videos on YouTube.

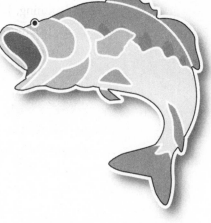

LARGEMOUTH BASS

Your little womb flopper is now the size of a sixteen-inch largemouth bass that weighs four to five pounds. Baby is hanging out in the live well. His sense of hearing is definitely heightened; he reacts to strange noises, especially the voice of the lady in Target asking your wife when the baby is due to arrive.

The amniotic sac has reached its maximum capacity of fluid by now. So what happens if Mommy's fish tank starts leaking in public? It probably won't be like a dam bursting but rather just a leak sprouting—especially if Nemo's in a head-down position. Imagine his noggin being used as a cork of sorts.

Once your little bass grows up a bit, you'll have the distinct joy of taking him fishing. Oh yes. Fishing! You probably have fond memories of when your own dad took you fishing. My dad took me fishing every summer, and every summer I would outfish my dad. The crazy thing is, I usually caught most of the fish on his line! I was that good, I guess.

Then I became a dad and took my own kids fishing. *What a different experience.* If you have yet to take kids fishing, let me break it down for you. You'll buy each of your kids a fishing rod, which will likely have some Disney character on it because that will be the one your kid wants. Pro tip: Buy the rods when you're at the store by yourself to avoid having to buy an Elsa tackle box. Elsa has some crazy magical powers, but none of them involve catching fish.

You'll finally arrive at the lake, and your kids will be excited. You'll carry all the gear from the truck as you chase after your kids, who are already standing on sharp rocks at the water's edge. This is where you'll start reciting "Don't Do That," the official dad chant of fishing:

Your kids are climbing the sharp rocks.
   "Don't do that."

Your kids are playing with the worms.
   "Don't do that."

Your kids are dumping out the tackle box.
   "Don't do that."

Your kids are swinging their rods like they're practicing a ribbon dance routine.
   "Don't do that."

Your kids are chasing the geese.
   "Don't do that."

You're now an hour into your angling excursion, and you have yet to cast your own line. Instead, you're untangling your kids' rods for the fifth time and explaining why they can't use the giant muskie lure with two treble hooks. "Daddy doesn't want any face piercings," you'll say. (Doesn't matter. You're going to get hooked sooner or later.) It's at this time that your kids will announce that they're bored and you'll do everything in your power to get even the tiniest bluegill on the line. You toss them a couple of juice boxes as you work to hook a six-inch fish. At this point you're not looking for a four-pound bass; you want quick, easy fish. If you want to hook your kids on fishing, you must first hook the fish for your kids!

Maybe you'll catch some fish, and maybe you won't. Either way, you'll go home exhausted and possibly defeated. Here's the encouraging part . . . They won't. They won't remember how many times you yelled, "Don't do that!" They won't remember you spending hours untangling their lines. They'll remember catching the one fish on your line—just like you did when you were a kid.

The best advice I was ever given about taking kids on adventures was from a dad I worked with on our TV show, *Super Dad*. His name is Andy, and he's an avid backpacker and all-around outdoorsman. When he and his wife started having kids, they made a commitment to keep backpacking while finding a way to take the kids along. They have hiked hundreds of miles with both babies and toddlers in tow. I asked him how he was able to do it without losing his mind. "Backpacking with kids? Do they bring their stuffed animals? Do you have to carry them most of the way? Do they complain half the time?"

His answer was simple: Lower your expectations. Don't plan to go ten miles; plan to go five. Take lots of snacks, play games, and find interesting things for them to look at along the way. You can't expect them to hike the way you used to and still have a good time. You'll have to adjust the experience to align with their interests and attention span.

I thought that was amazing advice. So as far as fishing goes, you won't be trying to catch a respectable four-pound bass; instead, you'll catch the easier four-ounce bluegill. But when your kid catches that four-ounce bluegill all by herself for the first time, it will be something you'll never forget. The smile on her face and the wonder in her eyes as she stares at the tiny catch will have you beaming. You'll soon realize that helping your kids experience something will bring you more joy than actually experiencing it yourself.

Then the reel on your daughter's *Frozen II* fishing rod will jam, and you'll curse Elsa under your breath.

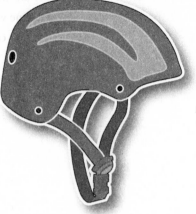

BICYCLE HELMET

Your child is now the size of a bicycle helmet, which *"you better darn well put on before you even think about touching that bike!"*

Does that sound familiar to you? Can you imagine yourself telling your kid this one day? Or maybe this is the last statement that would ever come out of your mouth.

There are two types of parents. The first makes sure their kid is wearing a bicycle helmet and kneepads and elbow pads and wrist guards and a reflective vest. The second type hucks their kid down an icy hill on nothing but an old piece of sheet metal full of rusty nails.

We love to put people into categories, don't we? Just think about the popularity of the Enneagram. "Oh, I totally can see that you're an Eight with a Seven wing! I'm a Three with a Two wing!" (Are these people speaking in code?) "I'm a Scorpio with an apple pie wing." *What is going on?* It's also fun and natural to put parents into specific categories. But when you break parenting into the major categories that people refer to today, like Lawnmower Parents and Tiger Parents, you'll find that there are strong qualities in all of them. The extremes are easy to lampoon, but many of these traits are rooted in a deep desire to love and nurture children well. So imagine what sort of dad you might become if you could cherry-pick the best of these types:

Lawnmower Dad is protective of his kid and mows down every hardship in her path. It makes for a smooth life . . . until Dad is no longer there to mow for her. "Daddy? Where's the pull start? How do I prime it?"

Helicopter Dad. A kid feels the wind from those helicopter blades as the dad hovers over him, getting involved in every aspect of his life. This is sort of like the Lawnmower Dad, but instead of mowing down all the adversity, he's just there to help with it . . . always watching from above.

Tiger Dad. Yes, you can be a Tiger Dad; this isn't solely reserved for moms. Tiger Woods's dad was both literally and figuratively a Tiger Dad. This is the dad who sets a high bar for his kid's academics and extracurricular activities, the type of parent who can produce an Olympic medalist or an astronaut (or a nervous basket case—be careful!).

Free-Range Dad gives his child copious amounts of freedom. No, he's not a neglectful parent but rather strives to make his kid independent and self-sufficient, challenging her to be able to get down from a tree on her own when no one is around to help. Let's just hope she doesn't break her shins.

Concierge Dad does everything he can to make his child's life on this planet a pleasant stay. It's less about what his kid needs and more about what his kid wants. "More towels? Coming right up, sir!"

Comic Dad lives life trying to make his child laugh, even at bedtime or when Mommy is frustrated, and might make a

living being funny on YouTube (hey . . . that sounds familiar).

Chameleon Dad changes his mood, methods, and manners
based on the social situation and what happens to be in
vogue at the time.

Career Dad is never there because he's so busy with work.

I'm one part Free-Range Dad, one part Comic Dad, and I usually
let my kids do their thing without much supervision. Maybe they're
climbing a tree and I'm looking from a distance to see if they're still
in it. Which one or ones are you likely to become? Are there any
changes you want to make when you think about the future? Or any
habits you want to double down on and intensify for the good of
your kiddos?

Parenting is about finding the middle ground or sweet spot in all
these slightly arbitrary categories. From there you can begin discovering tactics that suit your parenting style. There is a happy medium
that allows you to play with your kids and protect them. In reality
different moments may call for you to be a concierge, but a few minutes later, you're also needed as a chef and a chauffeur and a caretaker
and a carpenter and a counselor.

And when things get rough, remind your child that you're still the
CEO.

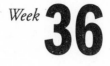

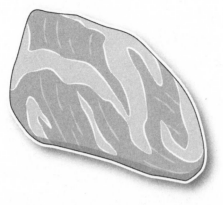

SIX-POUND BRISKET

Some say your baby by now is the size of a papaya or a bunch of kale. Really? Who wants to be compared to a tropical fruit or some leaf cabbage? Not me! And I can't imagine my epic little spawn does either. Let's set the record straight. Your baby is approximately the weight of a six-pound beef brisket and has been slow cooking inside Traeger-Mama for thirty-six weeks. Yes, that's a lot of baby, but most of his bones and cartilage remain soft so he can get through the birth canal. Your baby is also probably in a head-down position, getting ready to finally meet his parents for the first time. That's why they say, "Head up is breech, head down is brisket." I'm just kidding—they don't say that. Don't repeat that to the doctor. She'll think you're an idiot.

"Lightening" might strike your wife a few weeks before labor. This is what they call it when baby's head drops down into the pelvis. This lightens how the baby feels inside the womb, allowing them both a little more room to breathe. But a baby dropping also means Mom will have more pressure in her lower abdomen and may develop pelvic pain. Imagine walking around with a six-pound weight between your legs!

BONKERS FOR BRISKET

You ever notice that some dudes are a little too passionate about beef brisket? Especially the kind that's slow smoked for ten hours. Their lives revolve around that juicy, tender hunk of meat.

"Hey, man. You know what I'm doing this weekend?" your brisket-loving friend might ask you on a Friday afternoon.

His face will grow intense, as if he's about to tell you he's going to have open-heart surgery.

"What?"

"I'm making a brisket," he says, not as a response but rather as a declaration. You wait to hear something added to that, like he's making the brisket for an anniversary party or a family get-together, but no plan emerges other than his date with this big cut of beef.

"Yeah, it's pretty much gonna be my entire Saturday," he'll tell you. "I'm going to give it a dry rub tonight. I mix it with salt, pepper, brown sugar, onion and garlic powder, and chipotle seasoning. Then I'm gonna wake up at 4 A.M. to get the smoker going. That way the drum starts to reach temperature at exactly the right time." He says all this like it should be extremely interesting. This is where I usually like to ask him if he wants to borrow any of my Kraft barbecue sauce so I can watch him lose his brisket-lovin' mind.

This guy will spend all night thinking about the brisket, going over the schedule like a play-by-play in his mind. He'll clear out space in the fridge for this massive cut of meat to sit and marinate. He'll set an alarm to wake up in time to get the smoker going. He's likely putting more planning into preparing this hunk of brisket than he put into his own wedding.

Even before I had kids, I never found I wanted to spend that much time cooking up some cow. But some guys are bonkers about brisket. And more power to 'em, I guess. One of my best friends will tell me when he's going to be making a brisket. "Yeah, just got home from Costco. Got a brisket." Cool, bud. You bought some meat. Congrats.

Here's the thing: Nobody ever brags about buying some burgers at Costco. You don't spend hours working on a hamburger patty, marinating it the night before or smoking it or any of those things. You shouldn't cook a burger for seven to ten hours.

As much as I think my friends are nuts for getting up at 4 A.M. to start smoking fine meats, I can appreciate the dedication and effort. I guess being a dad is a bit like grilling. Are you going to be a brisket dad or a burger dad? Do you want to resemble someone who spends time planning, preparing, and making a brisket or someone who slaps some beef patties onto a grill, flips them once, and takes them off after ten minutes? I love a good burger as much as the next guy, but when it comes to parenting, quality work takes time and usually isn't convenient.

When you look ahead at becoming a father, try to picture giving your child the love and care that some guys give a brisket. Be an attentive father. Know what's happening with your child whatever age she's at, the same way someone might check a smoker and make sure it's set at the right temperature. Realize that teaching your kid is a lifelong process, one that's slow just like barbecuing in slow, dry heat. Sometimes you have to change directions as a parent, the same way you have to rotate the brisket every few hours. Don't get too hotheaded, but remain at a steady temperature; otherwise you might burn your relationship with your kid.

Okay, so this metaphor can go only so far, but you get what I'm talking about.

And don't even get me started on veggie burgers! Good night!

Parenting takes time and effort, but great parenting takes toil and sweat and tears and patience. And chipotle sauce.

Don't just go through the motions of being a dad. Be a brisket dad.

THIS WEEK

Chances are if you do end up making a brisket, your wife won't be able to eat much since the baby takes up so much room. So perhaps focus on lighter meals that you eat together more frequently. Save the hours you'd spend cooking up an actual brisket, and use those to help your wife with small but meaningful things. When she sits, try elevating her legs to help with her swollen feet and ankles. Or maybe schedule a pedicure for her.

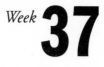

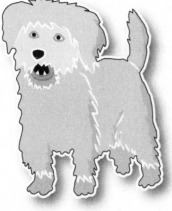

SMALL YIPPY DOG

The child curled up inside your lady is the size of a small yippy dog that you might see your neighbor walking down the street . . . So help me if she's *carrying* it in a purse! Thankfully for your wife, the baby's not getting much bigger, but his brain is growing like bonkers!

Your wife might start to experience Braxton-Hicks right about now too. Braxton-Hicks contractions are false labor pains. When a mother has them, she's not actually in labor yet; her body is just preparing for labor. It's the uterus's version of warming up the car on a cold morning. Not going anywhere just yet—just getting ready.

Now let's talk about that small yippy dog . . .

When I was in college, my brother and I bought this four-bedroom house and rented out the other two rooms. We rented one to this friend of ours who had this fluffy little thing she called a dog. Let me be clear, though: He was *not* what I consider to be a dog. Growing up in the country, we had four dogs at a time throughout my entire childhood. Labs, German shepherds, and rottweilers—dogs that could fetch, hunt, point, and even jump fences! You know, *real* dogs.

But our roommate didn't have a *real* dog. She had a generic small yippy dog. I don't remember the exact breed, but I'm pretty sure it was a mix of annoying and whiny.

This small yippy dog didn't know any tricks. He didn't listen to any commands. He wasn't even house-trained. He pooped all over our carpet on the regular. And he seemed to yip only when our roommate was gone. She would just leave the dog in her room while she was out doing whatever she was doing, and this small yippy dog would be in my basement—yipping.

One day I had a girl over to the house for a date, and I was making her an extravagantly prepared meal. At the time "extravagant" to me meant chicken alfredo, and I definitely made the sauce from scratch and didn't use the store-bought jar. That's a lie—I used the store-bought jar. But I warmed it up on the stove by myself! So I was in the middle of preparing this delicacy when the small yippy dog started doing what small yippy dogs do: He started yipping. My roommate wasn't home, and I assumed the dog just needed to be let outside, so I let the small yippy dog outside.

I left the dog alone for no more than two minutes while I tended to my date and my exquisite alfredo sauce, but when I returned, there was no small yippy dog. We didn't have a fence in the backyard, but why would that matter? I left him alone for only two minutes!

Alas, the small yippy dog was gone.

Now instead of enjoying our chicken alfredo, my date and I had to go wander around the neighborhood, looking for a small yippy dog that I didn't really want to find—calling out his name, hoping to hear him yip that yip that I hated. It was my roommate's dog, and for whatever reason, she loved that dog, so I needed to find him.

This, my friend, is what parenting is all about.

Parenthood is full of thousands of small yippy dogs. They're the things that are important to our kids but painfully annoying to us.

It's watching Blippi on your brand-new sixty-inch TV because your kid finds him more fascinating than NFL RedZone.

It's repouring your son's water because you gave him the red cup instead of the orange cup. (You monster!)

It's helping your daughter change her dress for the fourth time in one day because she's now in a purple mood.

It's the small battles that aren't worth fighting.

Every morning, you'll hear the small yippy dog while you're just trying to get out the door on time.

The small yippy dog might be your daughter telling you she needs you to get her stuffy after you've already buckled her into the car.

It might be your son waking up in the middle of the night, wailing about not being able to find his green Hot Wheels car.

Buddy, it's three in the morning. You don't need your green car. You need to go to sleep!

Of course, I don't say this, because he's in the zone where he's so worked up he can't listen to reason right now. He's also five and half awake. He just really needs to find his freaking green car, and I wouldn't recommend arguing with a five-year-old who doesn't have the ability to reason.

I'm going to go find his small yippy dog, which right now is his green car.

There are going to be moments when you have to put up with those small yippy dogs, when you have to go searching for them even though you really don't want to find them.

You do it because you love your child and because it gives him comfort.

As for what happened with my roommate's small yippy dog . . .

Unfortunately, we found him. Yippee ki yay!

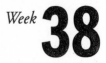
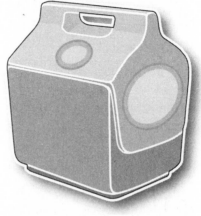

PLAYMATE LUNCH COOLER

Two more weeks! Give or take a week or two. How are you feeling? You got this! The clock is ticking and the countdown is underway. Right now the baby is nearly ready to go. Remember back in week 14 when I mentioned the baby's lanugo? What? You don't? That's okay— there isn't going to be a test at the end of this book. Lanugo is the fine hair that's been covering your baby. By now that's gone. So is most of the baby's vernix. Don't remember that either? Come on! Focus and go back to week 17. (Hint: It's more a sauce than fur.)

Your baby is now the size of a lunch cooler, the kind you might see next to a construction worker sitting way up on a steel beam four hundred feet in the air. Time and space are precious to him, so he has to pack the right meal for his short break. He gets a thirty-minute lunch break, and you know he's enjoying every minute of it before it's right back to work.

This reminds me of a truth I recently discovered as a dad. I was crazy busy working twelve-plus hours per day filming *Super Dad,* my TV series, while Heidi was back home with the kids all day. When I finally got home and walked through the door, Theo and Juno ran to me like I was Santa Claus, wanting to play Tickle Monster and have me chase them around the house forever. Then Theo and I played with these remote-controlled BattleBots before bedtime. Just before lights-out, Heidi asked Theo what his favorite part of the day was.

"Playing BattleBots with Dad!"

I could tell Heidi was a little bummed out by Theo's reply. Later that night, she told me why.

"You spent like twenty minutes playing BattleBots with him, and that was his favorite part of the day," she explained. "Meanwhile, I spent all day with him."

I realized that whichever parent spends less time with the kids often gets the opportunity to make a bigger impact in a shorter amount of time. Many times the working parent is a dad, and while I realize that isn't always the case, you're about to be a dad—so let's use that as an example. The kids have been waiting all day for you to get home, so when you do, they soak in the experience and relish every moment. Even though they've been learning from and playing with Mom all day long, they don't see that time as a precious resource. They're waiting for the couple of hours they'll have with *you* after you get home.

Think of it this way: You know those Starbucks Christmas cups, the ones they bring in every holiday season that make people think, *Oh yeah, here's the pretty, festive Christmas cup.* In reality it's a cup just like the other Starbucks cup. It doesn't necessarily work any better, and it doesn't make the coffee taste any better. But still, you get excited because you don't get to use a red cup that often. And that's what it's like when you get home after a long day! You're the Christmas cup.

Make sure you prioritize time with your kids, because it's *extremely* important to those little ones (and even the big ones). Kids will be acutely aware of the moments you're around . . . and they can tell whether or not they have your attention. So like the construction worker who has only thirty minutes to eat his ham sandwich from his Playmate cooler, make every minute count!

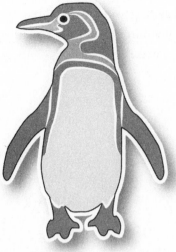

GALÁPAGOS PENGUIN

Your little nestling right now has reached his birth weight of six to eight pounds and is nineteen to twenty-two inches long, which just so happens to be the size of a Galápagos penguin! This type of penguin, the second smallest in the world, is unbelievably cute and lives north of the equator. It's also among the most endangered species of penguins.

Here's a cool fact about Galápagos penguins. They mate for life. These pint-size tuxedo-wearing creatures are role models for all married couples.

We can learn a lot from penguins. Emperor penguins live in Antarctica, and the males of this species spend seventy-five days in the dead of winter keeping their eggs warm while their wives are off at Penguin Target buying more throw pillows. Now, that's next-level parenting. They're some of the best dads in the animal kingdom.

Emperor penguins demonstrate how to be a truly great Dude Dad. Their journey into fatherhood begins rapidly: These penguins all converge on a particular meeting spot. Then they find their soul-mate in the midst of the thousands of penguins around them and decide to start a family. Some emperor penguins, however, start working on creating their offspring before it's time to cut the wedding cake! Chill, guys. Your grandmas are here . . .

Something marvelous and miraculous happens next. In the midst of extreme temperatures like fifty below zero, the female penguin lays a single fragile egg that needs to be kept warm. Mommy penguin then marches a long distance to the sea, where she'll gather food. So what does daddy penguin do? He steps up big time.

First the male emperor penguin carefully puts the egg on his feet to protect it from the frigid ice and under his belly to shield it from the bitter wind. Then he just stands there and waits for Mom to come back. "I'll be right back," she says, just like your wife tells you in the Target parking lot. But then she's gone for like seventy-five days. At least our hero is huddled up with other fathers doing the same thing. Just a bunch of awesome men, hanging out in the Target parking lot, caring for their eggs. Unfortunately, none of them know how to operate a propane grill, so they can't eat and they have to survive off their chunky dad bods.

Like us regular fathers, the male emperor penguin cares for the baby until Mom returns with milk and bread and lunch meat and candles and sandals. Before he can even check the receipt, Dad is sent to the sea to become the hunter-gatherer so Mom can feed the baby.

Yes, fathers are providers, but we're also nurturers. Penguins aren't the only ones who prove it. Now scientists are showing how men change when they become parents.

When my wife and I had our first two kids, she was working full time and I was working from home. So I got lots of one-on-one time with both of them. If you have the opportunity to do something like this, I highly recommend it. Your baby will be a baby for only a very short amount of time, and you both benefit so much from bonding with each other at this stage.

Did you know that women aren't the only ones who experience changes in their hormones and brain chemistry after having a baby? Men undergo these changes as well. Some studies find that men experience dips in their testosterone just before or after becoming a dad. While we don't know precisely why this occurs, the result is a more nurturing father. Instead of ripping their shirts and hulking out all the time, men can become more patient and loving. Studies suggest that lower levels of testosterone correspond with higher levels of oxytocin and dopamine in a dad's system as he bonds with and takes care of the new baby.

Some might think these traits make you less of a *man*. I think that's ridiculous. I say this makes you more of a well-rounded man. We can still be providers, use power tools, eat beef jerky, throw footballs, and wrangle steers while being nurturing to our babies. Those things aren't mutually exclusive. You can take a teeny tiny baby, hold her close, and bring her the comfort she needs to fall asleep. And just before she does, her big eyes will stare into yours as if you're her entire world. You may never feel like more of a man than in this moment.

PLAYLIST FOR GIVING BIRTH

When her water breaks . . .
"When the Levee Breaks" by Led Zeppelin

When her contractions have been four minutes apart and one minute long for one hour . . .
"4 Minutes" by Madonna, featuring Justin Timberlake and Timbaland

Driving your wife to the hospital . . .
"I Can't Drive 55" by Sammy Hagar

Arriving at the hospital . . .
"Doctor! Doctor!" by Thompson Twins

Waiting for the baby . . .
"You Can't Hurry Love" by the Supremes

Breathing techniques . . .
"Every Breath You Take" by the Police

Getting an epidural . . .
"Comfortably Numb" by Pink Floyd

Delivery (part 1) . . .
"Push It" by Salt-N-Pepa

Delivery (part 2) . . .
"I Want to Break Free" by Queen

Delivery (part 3) . . .
"Scream" by Michael Jackson

Holding your baby for the first time . . .
"Sweet Child o' Mine" by Guns N' Roses

For a son . . .
"Beautiful Boy (Darling Boy)" by John Lennon

For a daughter . . .
"Run the World (Girls)" by Beyoncé

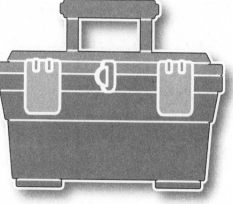

TOOLBOX

Use a screwdriver instead of a hammer. Try to untighten the nut with your hand. Utilize the path of least resistance first.

—TIM ALLEN

"Y'all ready for this?"

Cue the song "Get Ready," which you hear in every sporting arena and stadium.

"Nuh nuh nah nuna nuna, nuh nuh nah nuna nuna. Y'all ready for this?"

Bet you didn't know that this song comes from a Dutch music group called 2 Unlimited and that originally it was an instrumental track. See—this is why you read. You learn about the most important things in life.

It's almost go time. Things are about to get started. Right now your baby is the size of . . . a healthy newborn baby! But let's see if we can't come up with one final, memorable size object. I got it! This week, your little dude or dudette is the size of a toolbox. Which is certainly fitting since you're going to need a variety of tools as you enter this next phase of building a family.

DROPPING THE HAMMER

When you start out as a dad, you might have only a couple of tools at the ready, but you'll slowly acquire more and probably even borrow some from friends along the way.

Some tools will work for one situation but not for another. The hammer is a very useful tool. You can pound nails, you can pull nails, and you can bang things into place. But if you use your hammer to try to change your faucet . . . you're probably going to end up needing a new faucet. And some towels. A big part of maturing as a dad is being able to quickly identify the right tool for the job.

Some of the tools in my toolbox of dadhood actually came from my mom. She was great at individualizing her response to the child and situation at hand. One morning in my childhood stands out in my memory even now. On this particular day, I woke up in a bad mood—a very bad mood. I was determined to have a terrible, horrible, no-good, very bad day. I honestly don't remember why, but things weren't going my way, and they only kept getting worse. I ended up missing my bus, and Mom had to get me in the car and drive my grumpy butt to school. Mind you, we lived out in the country, so this was a seven-mile drive. I sat in the passenger seat with furrowed brow and tight lips. I was upset. I was pissed. I was being a little turd.

We rolled into town, and my mom did something unexpected. She drove right past the turn to my school. I looked over in confusion. *What's happening? Where are we going? Is she looking for a lake to throw me in?* Without saying a word, my mom kept going to our local doughnut shop and took me inside for a doughnut and chocolate milk. Now, this wasn't just any doughnut shop. This was Gary's Bakery. Gary's is known to have the best doughnuts in all of Miner County. They were considered a delicacy in our town of eight hundred people, and I was getting to miss school to enjoy one. I was speechless. I was grateful. I was apologetic. I can still taste that chocolate Long John with crushed peanuts and custard filling—my favorite.

Did I deserve a doughnut that day? Absolutely not. But my mom decided to show me grace and patience, and it turned my entire day around. She could have brought the hammer down on me, but instead, she reached a little deeper into her toolbox and pulled out the level. She stepped down into my world and helped level out all my topsy-turvy, off-kilter energy. She knew I was in a funk and needed some grace—and sugar—to get out of it. I arrived for school late that day but with a new attitude and a new appreciation for my mom.

CHECKMATE

As you develop as a dad, you may need to pick up some new tools from time to time. Dadhood is also going to force you to change some of your work habits.

Many men are task oriented. We're built to check boxes and get stuff done. I think it's why we bring in all the groceries in one trip. Car unloaded. Check. We crave that sense of accomplishment and completion. We're taught to go through life like this. You strive to get good grades so you can get into college. Check. Now you go to college and get that degree. Check. Now you use that degree to land your job. Check. Then you meet the girl of your dreams and know you need to marry her, so you get married. Check. Now you need to have three kids. Check. Check. Check! Here's the thing about our task lists, though. You can't check marriage and parenthood off some list. By definition, marriage and family aren't things you can ever be done with . . . not if you're in it for the long haul. You will never "complete" marriage. Marriage is an ongoing commitment that you have to continually invest in and work at, and so is parenting. They're not one-and-done things. They're things that continue to grow if you feed them and then in turn grow more and feed you.

My encouragement and challenge to you as you stand on the cusp of this grand adventure is to be less goal oriented and more process oriented. Take things slowly. Enjoy the journey of being a father rather than focusing on what you want to accomplish. *I want to take my kids to Disney. Okay, now I took them. Check!* Does it really matter if you check that very expensive Disney box? No. What's important is that you're spending time with your kids, whether they're riding Space Mountain or you're pushing them on a tree swing. It's about the experiences you're creating with them.

Marriage and parenting are grand adventures that you can't check off. What's important is the journey, not the result. That's because love is always growing. It's an action that we do but that thankfully is never done.

Being a dad is an experience that will never really end. It doesn't matter if your kid is eight or eighteen or thirty-eight; he's still going to need your love, guidance, and wisdom—you just have to express those things differently in different seasons of life. Even when your kid is grown and gone, your job isn't over; it simply takes on new forms. One day your kid may have his own kids. Then he'll be calling you to borrow some of his favorite tools from your toolbox. And you'll laugh at his struggles, knowing all too well what he's experiencing, because you've been there.

ACKNOWLEDGMENTS

Holy crap—I did it. I wrote a flippin' book! This is something that I dreamed of long before I ever knew what I would say. I can't tell you how incredibly thankful I am to have this opportunity to share my experiences and stories. It's now time to give credit where credit is due in making this all come to life.

First, I must thank my writing partner, Travis Thrasher, who selflessly watched all three hundred–plus videos I've ever made, panning for nuggets of gold within them. Thank you for the endless hours of Zoom calls and for teaching me that good books are not written with copious amounts of free time but are birthed out of the raw chaos of life.

To my editor and champion, Andrew, whose wife was pregnant while we were working on this book. You were by far the best subject to test this book on.

To my Dude Dad teammates, DJ and Berk, and both of your pregnant wives. I couldn't ask for better people to partner with not only in business but also in life.

To my parents for giving me not only examples to follow but also the freedom to try. Most of the parenting lessons I outline in this book I borrowed from your toolbox.

To my wife, Heidi. You don't just support everything I do—you elevate it. You are my rock.

To my kids. You will always be my greatest accomplishment, and all you have to do is be you. I love you.

SELECTED BIBLIOGRAPHY

Amato, Paula, and Maggie Blott, eds. *Pregnancy Day by Day: Count Down Your Pregnancy Day by Day with Advice from a Team of Experts and Amazing Images for Every Stage of Your Baby's Development.* Rev. ed. New York: DK, 2018.

Murkoff, Heidi. *What to Expect When You're Expecting.* 5th ed. New York: Workman, 2016.

Siegel, Daniel J., and Tina Payne Bryson. *No-Drama Discipline: The Whole-Brain Way to Calm the Chaos and Nurture Your Child's Developing Mind.* New York: Bantam Books, 2016.

Siegel, Daniel J., and Tina Payne Bryson. *The Whole-Brain Child: 12 Revolutionary Strategies to Nurture Your Child's Developing Mind.* New York: Bantam Books, 2012.

Wick, Myra J. *Mayo Clinic Guide to a Healthy Pregnancy.* Rev. ed. Rochester, Minn.: Mayo Clinic, 2018.

NOTES

WEEK 2: SPERM

The first epigraph is taken from Paula Amato and Maggie Blott, eds., *Pregnancy Day by Day: Count Down Your Pregnancy Day by Day with Advice from a Team of Experts and Amazing Images for Every Stage of Your Baby's Development,* rev. ed. (New York: DK, 2018), 42.

release about 250 million sperm: "Sperm Count and Pregnancy Rates," WINFertility, www.winfertility.com/blog/sperm-count-pregnancy-rates.

killed by flesh-eating bacteria: "24 Things That Are More Likely to Happen Than Winning the Lottery," MoneyMiniBlog, https://moneyminiblog.com/lists/things-more-likely-happen-winning-lottery.

killed by a meteorite: Lonnie Shekhtman, "How Likely Are You to Get Hit by a Meteor?," *Christian Science Monitor,* February 9, 2016, www.csmonitor.com/Science/Spacebound/2016/0209/How-likely-are-you-to-get-hit-by-a-meteor.

eleven fingers or toes: Rebekah Kuschmider, "What to Know About Polydactyly," WebMD, November 9, 2021, www.webmd.com/children/what-to-know-polydactyly.

injured by a toilet: Sarah Long, "17 Random Statistics That Will Actually Surprise You," SheKnows, May 3, 2018, www.sheknows.com/living/articles/1023453/what-are-the-odds-21-statistics-that-will-surprise-you.

WEEK 5: MATCH HEAD

miscarriage is around 20 percent: Zawn Villines, "What Are the Average Miscarriage Rates by Week?," Medical News Today, September 26, 2021, www.medicalnewstoday.com/articles/322634.

1 percent chance of a miscarriage: "Miscarriage Probability Chart," Datayze, https://datayze.com/miscarriage-chart.

WEEK 6: KERNEL OF POPCORN

"love hormone": Micah Toub, "The Science of How Fatherhood Transforms You," *Today's Parent,* June 8, 2021, www.todaysparent.com/family /parenting/the-science-of-how-fatherhood-transforms-you.

WEEK 8: TEN-MILLIMETER SOCKET

250,000 cells per minute: Sandra Ackerman, *Discovering the Brain* (Washington, D.C.: National Academies Press, 1992), chap. 6, www.ncbi.nlm .nih.gov/books/NBK234146.

People call this wonderful invention: Dana Dubinsky, "172 Pet Names for the Pacifier," BabyCenter, www.babycenter.com/baby/crying-colic/172 -pet-names-for-the-pacifier_3659111.

WEEK 14: TAPE MEASURE

body hair called lanugo: Heidi Murkoff, *What to Expect When You're Expecting,* 5th ed. (New York: Workman, 2016), 212.

actually "to teach": Ken Ginsburg, "What Does Discipline Really Mean?," The Center for Parent and Teen Communication, September 4, 2018, https://parentandteen.com/what-does-discipline-really-mean.

WEEK 15: BEER CAN

Your baby's eyes: Kate Marple, "15 Weeks Pregnant," BabyCenter, April 13, 2021, www.babycenter.com/pregnancy/week-by-week/15-weeks-preg nant.

WEEK 16: GRENADE

Die Hard: Die Hard, directed by John McTiernan (Century City, Calif.: Twentieth Century Fox, 1988).

WEEK 17: BOTTLE OF SANITIZER

vernix caseosa: Heidi Murkoff, *What to Expect When You're Expecting,* 5th ed. (New York: Workman, 2016), 246.

half as much time: "Children Spend Only Half as Much Time Playing

Outside as Their Parents Did," *The Guardian,* July 27, 2016, www.the
guardian.com/environment/2016/jul/27/children-spend-only-half-the
-time-playing-outside-as-their-parents-did.

because of the clean environment: Jacqueline Britz, "Can Cleanliness
Increase the Risk of Allergies and Asthma?," National Center for Health
Research, www.center4research.org/can-cleanliness-increase-risk-allergies
-asthma.

WEEK 21: QUART OF OIL

The epigraph is taken from *Seinfeld,* season 6, episode 19, "The Fusilli
Jerry," directed by Andy Ackerman, created by Larry David and Jerry
Seinfeld, aired April 27, 1995, on NBC.

WEEK 23: BOSE NOISE-CANCELING HEADPHONES

55 percent of all face-to-face communication: "How Much of Communication Is Nonverbal?," The University of Texas Permian Basin, https://
online.utpb.edu/about-us/articles/communication/how-much-of
-communication-is-nonverbal.

"get what you want": The Rolling Stones, "You Can't Always Get What You
Want," by Keith Richards and Mick Jagger, *Let It Bleed,* London Records,
1969.

WEEK 24: CONCESSION-STAND NACHOS

born at twenty-four weeks: "Obstetric Care Consensus No. 6: Periviable
Birth," *Obstetrics & Gynecology* 130, no. 4 (October 2017), https://jour
nals.lww.com/greenjournal/Abstract/2017/10000/Obstetric_Care
_Consensus_No__6__Periviable_Birth.57.aspx.

WEEK 28: MILK JUG

two hundred to five hundred extra calories: Donna Murray, "Breastfeeding
and the Calories You Eat," Verywell Family, April 20, 2020, www.very
wellfamily.com/how-many-extra-calories-does-a-breastfeeding-mom
-need-431858.

WEEK 29: HUMAN HEAD

triple in weight: Kate Marple, "29 Weeks Pregnant," BabyCenter, July 22, 2020, www.babycenter.com/pregnancy/week-by-week/29-weeks-preg nant.

"It's alive!": *Frankenstein,* directed by James Whale, Universal Pictures, 1931.

WEEK 30: GARBAGE DISPOSAL

fastest-selling books: "Richard Carlson: Bestselling Self-Help Guru," *The Independent,* December 30, 2006, www.independent.co.uk/news/obitu aries/richard-carlson-430230.html.

"I've never met anyone": Richard Carlson, *Don't Sweat the Small Stuff . . . and It's All Small Stuff: Simple Ways to Keep the Little Things from Taking Over Your Life* (New York: Hyperion, 1997), 62.

WEEK 39: GALÁPAGOS PENGUIN

Galápagos penguins: "Galápagos Penguin," Animalia, https://animalia.bio /galapagos-penguin.

Emperor penguins: "Emperor Penguin Breeding Cycle," Australian Antarctic Program, www.antarctica.gov.au/about-antarctica/animals/penguins /emperor-penguins/breeding-cycle.

how men change: Anna Machin, "How Men's Bodies Change When They Become Fathers," *The New York Times,* April 15, 2020, www.nytimes .com/2020/04/15/parenting/baby/fatherhood-mens-bodies.html.

dips in their testosterone: Machin, "How Men's Bodies Change."

WEEK 40: TOOLBOX

The epigraph is taken from Tim Allen, "What I've Learned: Tim Allen," interview by Cal Fussman, *Esquire,* August 27, 2011, https://classic .esquire.com/article/2011/11/1/tim-allen.

"Get Ready,": 2 Unlimited, "Get Ready," *Get Ready!,* Byte Records, 1992.

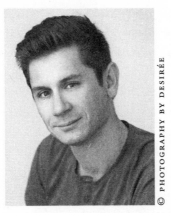

Actor and comedian Taylor Calmus, more frequently known as Dude Dad, parodies everyday family life through comedy sketches, vlogs, and DIY videos. His videos have entertained millions on social media and taught men everywhere how to be a dude even while changing a diaper. Calmus also stars on the Magnolia Network's *Super Dad,* in which he helps other dads make their kids' backyard dreams a reality.

Calmus is originally from the rural community of Howard, South Dakota, where he grew up building BMX ramps and learning the value of hard work. He spent ten years in Los Angeles, where he appeared in numerous TV shows and commercials and made numerous appearances on *Jimmy Kimmel Live!* Calmus now lives in Colorado with his wife, Heidi, and their children.